LOVE ME!

Marianne Power is a journalist and the author of the global bestseller *Help Me!*. Published in twenty-five languages, Marianne's wry, funny, down-to-earth and moving exploration of self-help books captured the world's imagination. *Love Me!* is her second book.

Also by Marianne Power

Help Me!

Marianne Power

LOVE ME!

One woman's search for a different happy ever after

PICADOR

First published 2024 by Picador
an imprint of Pan Macmillan
The Smithson, 6 Briset Street, London EC1M 5NR
EU representative: Macmillan Publishers Ireland Ltd, 1st Floor,
The Liffey Trust Centre, 117–126 Sheriff Street Upper,
Dublin 1, D01 YC43
Associated companies throughout the world
www.panmacmillan.com

ISBN 978-1-5290-5788-1 HB
ISBN 978-1-5290-5789-8 TPB

1 3 5 7 9 8 6 4 2

A CIP catalogue record for this book is available from the British Library.

Typeset in Dante by Jouve (UK), Milton Keynes
Printed and bound by CPI Group (UK) Ltd, Croydon, CR0 4YY

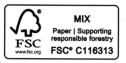

Visit **www.picador.com** to read more about all our books
and to buy them. You will also find features, author interviews and
news of any author events, and you can sign up for e-newsletters
so that you're always first to hear about our new releases.

'Your task is not to seek for love, but merely to seek and find all the barriers within yourself that you have built against it.'   *Rumi*

'You only have to let the soft animal of your body / love what it loves'   *Mary Oliver*

'I always thought you'd suit being a nun.'   *Mum*

Me: About this book.

Mum: Yes?

Me: There's going to be sex in it – is that OK with you?

Mum: Write whatever you want, Marianne!

Me: Good. I was worried I'd embarrass you.

Mum: But you're not writing about yourself again, are you?

Me: Yes.

Mum: Don't you think people have had enough of that?

Contents

LOVE ME!

A Happy Ending Makes for a Crap Beginning

'He didn't show up.'

'What do you mean he didn't show up?'

'I mean he wasn't there, at the airport.'

'Did you call him?'

'He didn't pick up.'

'Oh, Marianne. I'm sorry. Where are you now? James – wait, please! I'm on the phone. Sorry . . .'

'It's OK. I'm at the Airbnb.'

'Is it nice at least?'

I looked around the apartment for the first time. There were a lot of hard surfaces. 'I'm worried. What if something's happened to him? His dad was really sick last time we spoke and he was getting chest pains.'

'The Greek had chest pains or the dad?'

'The Greek. I think it's stress. He has a new job and is caring for both his parents and not sleeping and—'

'I'm sure he's OK – James, what is it? If you're hungry, have a satsuma – sorry.'

'It's OK, I should let you go.'

'So what are you going to do now?'

'I dunno. Wait to hear from him I guess.'

Gemma hung up and I walked to the French doors that looked onto the glistening lights of Athens.

I waited for the excitement I usually felt when arriving in a new city. It didn't come. I walked around the apartment, into the giant bedroom and two bathrooms. Its size felt like an affront. I shouldn't be here alone. This was a place for a couple.

What if something had happened to him? What if he'd had a heart attack?

I walked into the kitchen. There was a welcome basket on the counter, filled with fruit and a bottle of wine. My heart lifted at the sight of the wine. All was not lost. I could have a nice drink, sit on the balcony and wait for him to call.

I opened the drawers looking for a corkscrew but couldn't find one.

I wondered if it was too desperate to smash open the bottle.

Then another thought landed: what if this whole thing was pretend? What if he had no intention of meeting me? What if my love interest didn't live in Athens with his parents? What if he lived here with his wife and children?

Oh my god, was I being catfished?

I looked at the wine. I couldn't smash it. That would be a step too far.

I wheeled my suitcase to the bedroom. I took off my clothes and lay on the bed in my underwear, switching on my laptop. I fell asleep watching *Sneaky Pete*.

The next morning, I checked my phone. No messages.

I checked Instagram and scrolled through old posts. I stopped on one from a photo shoot with *Elle* magazine in Paris. I was standing in front of a painted backdrop in a little attic in the Marais blinking into the camera, stunned by my circumstances.

The book I'd written about my year-long quest to improve my life by following the rules of self-help had been published around the world, and I'd spent the previous months getting on planes, trains and automobiles to promote it. I was interviewed on Polish daytime telly, before a segment on crystal litter boxes. I was flown to New York where I appeared on morning television after Martha Stewart. I'd spoken to hundreds of ravers coming down at a festival in Holland and to a room full of farmers in the west of Ireland.

Before the Paris photoshoot, I'd been interviewed by a woman who looked like Isabella Rossellini. Drinking coffee on plump velvet armchairs in a hotel bar she told me she loved the book. She could relate to it, she said. I was flattered. And confused. How could a woman with such perfect nails relate to my insecurities or hangovers?

I had spent the interview mesmerized by her dancing hands.

On her left hand she was wearing two rings stacked together, with purple and orange stones. I asked her where she'd got them and she said a name that meant nothing to me. 'It is not a shop where you buy for yourself – you must get a man to buy it for you.' She smiled knowingly and I smiled back, acting like this was also the world I inhabited, a world where men bought me expensive jewellery.

She leaned forward. 'Perhaps the Greek will buy it for you?' she suggested. 'Did you see him again?'

And there it was – the question everybody got to eventually: what happened to the Greek?

I'd done so much in the name of self-improvement. I'd modelled naked, jumped out of a plane, chatted to strangers on the tube and even planned my own funeral. I'd had moments of enlightenment and bliss. Epiphanies and crises.

And yet, despite all the profound learnings and Buddha-like growth, all anyone wanted to know was what had happened to the tall, dark, handsome stranger I met in the coffee shop along the way.

At the start of the project a friend had joked that the whole thing would have been a failure if it didn't end with a boyfriend. I was so angry at this outdated idea that happiness had to come in the form of a man, and told her so. And yet, part of me thought maybe she was right.

'Well, actually . . .' I said, also leaning forward towards the French journalist. 'I'm flying to Athens next week to see him.' She smiled again and I leaned back, delighted that for once I was not the single loser. I was part of a love story!

This was a new experience for me. At the age of forty I had spent most of my life single. In my teens and twenties, I thought the problem was that I was unattractive and nobody wanted me . . . I was too ginger, too fat, too . . . whatever it was, I was not the kind of girl guys liked.

In my thirties, I discovered that some guys *did* like me, but I struggled to stay with them for more than a few months. Then I told myself that my problem was not that I was unattractive, it was that I hadn't met the right man.

At thirty-six, I went to an intense therapy week called the Hoffman Process, where I found myself standing in front of twenty-five strangers telling them that I didn't think anyone decent would love me. I hadn't known I'd thought that until I was saying it. Then I thought, maybe I've been repelling love because I don't think I deserve it.

After all the self-help, I felt much better in myself.

And then I met the Greek.

I'd met him while trying a masochistic form of self-help called Rejection Therapy, which involves getting rejected by another human every single day for a month. The idea is that by actively seeking out rejection, you get used to it and the feeling of crushing humiliation and failure. Once you get used to this, the theory goes, you can go forth and conquer life, without being held back by the fear of hearing 'no'.

The month had not gone well. I'd smiled at strangers on the underground, which is something they'll arrest you for in London. I asked for free coffees only to be given a half-hour breakdown of how bad business was by my local coffee-shop owner. For one horrifying week I prepared to audition for *The X Factor*. Then my uncle died and I was saved by a funeral.

A few days after the funeral I walked into a coffee shop in Soho and spotted a hot guy I'd seen there months before. The first time I'd seen him I'd been so struck by his beardy loveliness I'd told my friend Rachel about him. She'd said I should have said hello, and I scoffed. I didn't say hello to men I fancied. Instead, my approach was to imagine all the ways that I was not good enough for the object of my affection while looking in any direction but theirs.

But this month was different. I had to say hello to him and face my deepest fear: rejection from a handsome man.

For four hours – I'm not exaggerating – I watched him write while I pretended to work. Sometimes he'd catch me looking at him and I'd look away in a hot panic. Then his friend joined him and I walked out, kicking myself for the missed opportunity and for being such a loser. Why was I so shit with men? Why? When would this ever change?

I crossed the street to go to the work drinks but just as I was given a glass of warm Prosecco to celebrate the launch of a new mattress – booze and beds, a fitting representation of my comfort zone – I told my colleague I had to go. I walked right back across the road, into the coffee shop and up to his table. The two dark-haired men looked up at me. I looked down.

'Hello,' I said but hadn't thought any further than that.

'I was just leaving, would you like my seat?' the friend asked me, like it was the most normal thing on earth.

'Would you like a coffee?' my beardy crush asked.

'Yes please.'

We drank coffee and chatted easily and he asked if I'd like to go for a glass of wine. He walked me to my train and kissed me on the platform. He told me that me walking up to him was one of the nicest things that had happened to him.

Then he flew back to Athens, where he cared for his sick parents.

Since then we'd spoken regularly, long Skype sessions into the night. He'd come to London for a few days and we agreed that when my book was published, I would hand deliver it to Athens. 'I want to see your name on the cover and smell the pages. I can't wait for that day,' he said. Here I was. So where was he?

My phone beeped. I grabbed it. A message from Rachel, with two emojis (an aubergine, a heart) and three question marks.

'Do you think he'll be waiting at the airport with flowers?' she'd asked before I left. The thought hadn't occurred to me. No man had ever met me at an airport before, let alone with flowers.

'Did you get sexy underwear?' she asked.

'No!' I snapped, embarrassed.

I had. From Liberty. Two sets: black and sky blue. They were see-through and very not me. The knickers had a peephole in the back and the bra squashed my nipples. It made my boobs look like they were being held hostage. But maybe that was sexy? Standing in the carpeted changing room, I worried that my tummy was hanging over the knickers, but then I remembered that I was meant to be too enlightened to think this way.

I bought them and imagined wearing them in bed while the sun set on the terrace, a gentle wind floating through white gauzy curtains . . . his fingers tracing the outline of my body . . .

Trust me to run off into the sunset with someone who didn't show up.

He did show up in the end. Well, a day later. Sweating and panting by the door. It was 9 p.m. and I'd spent twenty-four hours walking around a hot and dusty Athens, hating every ancient rock and smiling couple.

'I thought you said the fourteenth,' he said, breathless in the stairwell. I was on the fifth floor and the lift wasn't working.

'I said the twelfth,' I said, staring at the marble floor.

'I wrote down the fourteenth. Babe, I'm so sorry.'

'I tried calling you, I Skyped you like ten times,' I told the floor.

'I don't have Skype on my cell and I haven't been at home – dad got taken to hospital again.'

I looked up from the floor. The circles under his eyes were black.

'I'm sorry,' I said. 'Is he OK?'

'He's hanging in there,' he said with a shrug.

I pulled the door open and he walked into the apartment.

He came in for a hug. 'I have strep throat . . . so I cannot even kiss you,' he said.

'That's OK,' I said. It wasn't OK.

He started asking me about what I'd been doing and was the flight OK and I could see it was taking every ounce of energy for him to keep talking.

'I'm sorry,' he said again. 'That I wasn't there at the airport. This was not what I imagined.'

'It's OK,' I said. And this time it was OK.

'We don't need to talk. Why don't you rest?' I said.

We moved to the sofa and he rested his head on my legs as I stroked his hair.

Within minutes he was asleep.

I switched on the television, which had Netflix, and watched some high-school movie quietly. Near the end of the movie, he woke up with a start.

'What time is it?'

I looked at my phone. It was past eleven.

He jumped up from the sofa. 'I shouldn't have slept. I need to get back to mum. She is at home on her own. I'm so sorry.'

He put on his jacket and looked around the room.

'Did I bring a bag?' he asked, almost frantic.

'No, I don't think so.'

'OK, I need to go,' he looked haunted. 'Every time I leave them I think something will happen.'

For the next three days I wandered around the city on my own.

We met a couple of times, when he would spend half an hour with me before sprinting back to his parents or work.

I googled things to do in Athens and found a quote from Don DeLillo, who described the Acropolis as looming above the traffic 'like some monument to doomed expectations'.

On the flight home I asked myself the questions I'd asked myself a million times: what was wrong with me? Why didn't these things ever work out for me? You know – love things. Why couldn't I do this thing that everyone around me seemed to do? Meet someone, fall in love, and all the stuff that went with it?

I waited in the rain for an Uber to pick me up from City airport. Despite the weather, I felt relieved to be home.

I was lucky, I told myself.

I was not the one caring for two sick parents, living off next to no sleep. So my romantic adventure hadn't gone to plan, but that was OK. My life was still good.

The silver Prius pulled up and I jumped in.

'Marann-y?' he asked.

'Yes.'

'E5?'

'Yes, please.'

We got onto the road and drove past roadworks, cranes and police cars. I was looking forward to getting back to my own flat, my own bed and my own life. I would pretend this whole trip hadn't happened.

'Been anywhere nice?' my driver asked.

'Greece.'

'Holiday?'

'I was visiting a friend.'

'Was it hot?'

'Warm.'

'Rain here.'

'Yeah, I can see.'

I turned my head and looked at pictures of small children dangling from his rear-view mirror; little chubby faces grinning with missing teeth. I smiled.

'You have children?' the driver asked.

'No.'

'You have a boyfriend? Husband?'

'No.'

'How old are you?'

'Forty.'

'Forty!'

'Yes, forty.'

'I thought you were young—'

I smiled at the kind-of-compliment.

'But you are not!'

Oh.

'You must find a husband and have children! They will look after you when you are old. My children – they buy me presents. They visit me. They have children now and my grandchildren make me very happy!'

'That's nice – but not everyone—'

'So why no husband?'

'I—'

Before I could mount a defence of my life choices, he was pulling into my road.

'Please, you go quick – there is someone behind me!'

And with that I was left literally and metaphorically on the kerb.

I spent the next day in bed watching serial killers, ignoring messages from friends asking how it had gone. I wished I hadn't told everyone. I wished I hadn't – literally – alerted the international media.

Lying in bed, watching women be decapitated in supermarket car parks on my dirty laptop screen, old feelings flooded my body. Feelings of shame, rejection and inadequacy.

I felt humiliated.

'You didn't even get a kiss?' asked Rachel, when I called her back.

'Nope.'

'No shagging?'

'None. Seriously. The poor guy had a flu, was working all hours and then running to see his dad in the hospital and caring for his mum at home.'

'Are you disappointed?' she asked.

I thought about it.

'Yes, but mostly I felt guilty that I put him under pressure to see me when he had so much going on.'

'But I thought that was what you'd agreed?' asked Rachel. 'That you'd go with the book.'

'It was, but I knew the timing wasn't right and I pretty much made him say it was OK for me to come.'

'I'm sure you didn't.'

'No really, I did.'

I cringed to admit it, even to myself, but the truth was he hadn't been getting back to me when I suggested visiting – but I booked it anyway and told him I knew other people in Athens, so it would be great if we could meet up but there was no pressure.

'*Do* you know other people in Athens?' Rachel asked.

'No.'

'Oh.'

'Yeah. It wasn't fair on him. It was selfish.'

'It's not selfish to want to see someone you like. I'd love someone to get on a plane to see me.'

'Yeah, but . . .' I tried to find the words for something I'd been struggling to understand myself. 'I don't know how much I really wanted to see him or how much I thought I should see him because . . . well, that's what I was meant to be doing.'

'But I thought you liked him?'

'I do! I really do! He is one of the kindest, smartest men I've ever met, but he's just a man I met in a coffee shop . . .

then I wrote about him and everyone kept asking about him, and I think . . . I went to see him because . . . well, I was trying to play out some happy-ever-after fantasy.'

'So you're not heartbroken?' she asked.

I thought about it. I felt guilty that I'd put him under pressure. Embarrassed about yet another romantic failure. But heartbroken . . . ?

'I mean, I wanted to see him and have a nice time, but I don't know. It wasn't like I ever saw us being together for ever . . .'

Just the phrase 'together for ever' made me want to scratch my skin off. A prison, not a prize. Even with someone as lovely as the Greek.

'Do you actually want a relationship?' she asked.

I paused.

'I don't know. I know I'm supposed to want one but it just doesn't seem to work out for me. I think maybe it's just not for me.'

'Don't say that!' she said, like it was the worst thing ever. 'You can't give up just because one thing didn't work out. It hasn't exactly worked out for me, but I keep trying.'

And she did. Dating was the part-time job she did on top of her full-time job. She was so sure she wanted to meet someone and have a family, and she was doing whatever it took. I wasn't sure about any of it.

Why did I seem to be so ambivalent about this thing that everybody else was so sure about? Why, aged forty, had I not had any relationships that lasted for more than a few months?

Had I just not met the right guy? Or was I deeply messed up in some way that I didn't understand? Did I have intimacy issues that I needed to work through? Did I just feel this way because I hadn't experienced true love and therefore didn't know what I was missing? Or was it, maybe, something else?

1

Single at Heart

'I never thought you'd get married,' said mum. 'Don't you remember, I said that to you when you were a teenager and your dad got annoyed at me.'

'Oh, yeah.' I could picture it straight away. My sisters and I were at the kitchen table asking mum what she thought we'd be when we grew up.

'I don't think you'd like the domesticity, you'd feel trapped,' said mum now, at a different kitchen table but next to the same teapot.

'Yeah, but it's not like that any more. I could be with a guy who does the cooking and cleaning – or we could pay someone to do it.'

Mum scoffed. Both, presumably, at the idea of a man cooking and cleaning, and at paying someone to do what you can do yourself.

'Don't you want me to get married?' I asked. 'Most parents want their kids to get married.'

'I want you to be happy, that's all.'

'But you got married.'

'Your father was the last person on earth I expected to meet. He was a complete one-off and that was that. I could just as easily not have married. It was never important to me. You just have to live your life, do what you want to do, and if you meet someone – great, and if you don't, that's fine too.'

'But the whole "going off into the sunset" thing, it's in all the books and films and songs as the point of life. It's what all my friends are doing—'

'Not all of them.'

'OK, most of them . . . If I don't get married, will I be missing the point of life?' I asked.

'Oh, for God's sake, Marianne.'

'I'm serious.'

'You live a charmed life.'

'I know.'

'You have a freedom that most people would die for.'

'I know.'

'And you have so many friends.'

'I know, but I get lonely.'

'You can be married and lonely. The idea that you meet someone and it's going to be this blissful state – that's not how it is. And it's not in your control whether you meet someone – if it's going to happen, it'll happen.'

'You can help your chances by dating.'

'So do that then.'

'I don't want to.'

'Well, then. Maybe you don't want what you don't have.'

On the walk home I thought about what she'd said. Could it be that simple? That I didn't want what I didn't have?

Almost everything else in life I'd wanted, I'd been fortunate enough to get. I'd written a book, I'd travelled the world. I'd met so many interesting people. If I really wanted to fall in love and settle down, surely I'd have done it by now?

So why did I doubt myself so much?

Because it was lonely and confusing not to be doing what ninety per cent of the people around me were either doing or trying to do. Because even today a woman's greatest achievements are still considered to be partnership and children.

To be a single, childless woman at forty was to have got life wrong. Even Uber drivers knew that.

I walked past my local pub. People were smoking outside, jittering with Saturday night hopes. The women looked cold in heels and low-cut tops and a table of lads were hunched over their drinks pretending not to look at them. The door opened and I could hear the dull roar of people's voices bouncing on hardwood floors.

My first thought was: 'You'd have to pay me to go in there.' Then another voice said, 'You should go in, it's a Saturday night . . . You never know who you'll meet.'

But I never met men in pubs – did anyone? – and I was tired of going through life thinking I should keep the door open to someone new. Keeping the door open was causing a draft. Couldn't I just close it?

And yet, as soon as I said that to myself another voice said, 'You're just fooling yourself. In denial. Of course you want to meet somebody. Of course you do. Everybody does.'

I got to the chip shop opposite my flat and hovered.

A bit of me worried that people would judge a single woman buying chips on a Saturday night. 'Look at her, fat cow, nothing else for company but a bag of chips. She'll never meet someone if she keeps eating like that . . .'

I went in and ordered a small bag before crossing the road to my building.

The guy downstairs had Phil Collins on loudly. I could smell damp and weed.

I turned on my light and smiled to remember that I'd cleaned. Well, that's a lie. Anne had cleaned. My rented flat was the size of two-and-a-half postage stamps, and I had a cleaner. Mum was right, domesticity was not my strength. Anne came once a month and I liked chatting to her about her four kids, her nieces and nephews in Ireland and her sister, who is a devotee of the law of attraction.

She looked at my tiny flat like it was a piece of heaven. 'I'd live here quite happily,' she'd say, rubber gloves on. 'Nobody can get you up here, nobody wants anything from you.' She was a woman who had spent her whole life looking after other people. Like mum.

I looked at my dining-table-cum-desk, sitting by a window with papers and flowers on it. That was always my dream: a desk by a window with flowers on it. Somewhere I could sit and write and think and watch the world go by.

And I had it.

I ate the chips from the bag.

When I finished, I pulled out the magnifying mirror and spent a happy ten minutes squeezing blackheads before retiring to bed with *Grace and Frankie*.

As I pulled the duvet up to my neck, I could hear the couple next door arguing. I turned the volume up and wondered how Lily Tomlin looked so good. And how much work did it take to make her curly hair look that naturally perfect? Was it a wig?

It was 9 p.m. on a Saturday night and I was alone in bed watching a show about two pensioners. That was sad, wasn't it?

So why was I quite happy?

Sunday morning and I woke up with mum's phrase still in my head. *Maybe you don't want what you don't have.* I turned it over like a penny. Over and over and over. It was a relief to allow it as a possibility. If I didn't want what I didn't have, I could stop treating the life that I had now as this temporary limbo before the real thing started.

I got out of bed and went into the kitchen to put the kettle on. As it boiled, I stood by the window and looked out at the market stalls that pitch up on my street on the weekend. It was like a Richard Curtis version of London, but with more hoods and hipsters.

I looked down at couples deciding between succulents at the flower stall. I imagined them bringing them back to their flats, before cooking a roast and watching a film on the sofa. Surely I wanted that too?

I thought about it.

Not particularly.

Maybe *this* was what I wanted? My life as it was. Single, in a tiny flat, with a desk, a window and flowers. But was that sad? Giving up?

I decided to ask the all-knowing gods of Silicon Valley. I made coffee, sat down at my laptop and typed into Google: 'Can you be happy and single?'

A string of articles came up with titles such as Yes, Single People Can Be Happy and Healthy! and Nine Ways Being Single Can Improve Your Life.

I started clicking.

One argued that single people are thinner than those in a relationship. Apparently people gain on average fourteen pounds when they couple up. Another suggested that it was good to be single rather than with someone who spends all your money. (It didn't explain what to do when you're single and you spend all your money.)

The articles were illustrated with photos of women doing yoga on a beach and splayed out in a starfish position on the bed. The message seemed to be: you might be single, but you are also super cute and sexy and will find someone soon . . . just keep doing that yoga!

Some even said as much. They made the point that being single was a great time to get to know yourself, which would then help you know who was right for you. They reminded me that I had to love myself first, before I could welcome love in from another.

Nothing I read seemed to be suggesting that it would be OK to be single for ever.

But then I came across a TEDx Talk by a woman called Bella DePaulo entitled, 'What no one ever told you about people who are single.'

I clicked on it and saw a grey-haired woman stand on stage and announce to the crowd, 'I'm sixty-three, and I have been single my whole life!'

She said it in the same tone of voice in which she'd say, 'I'm sixty-three and I've won the lottery!' I'd never seen someone talk with such positivity about being single. It felt radical.

DePaulo kept smiling as she talked about how, in her twenties and thirties, she knew she was supposed to get married and that she was supposed to want to get married, but . . . well, she never did. Do it, or want to.

As she put it: 'Everything about my life had led up to a different story – that being single was my happy ever after.'

Wow. Was that even an option?

DePaulo had the same doubts. She questioned herself, because 'positive, affirming stories about single life have never been part of our lives the way fairy tales have.'

She made it her mission to find those stories. She feared that studies would show that, just like the fairy tales, being in a couple made you happier and healthier. But they didn't prove that – not at all.

After analysing 800 studies, DePaulo found that people are not made happier by getting married. They might experience a short peak of happiness around their wedding but they soon revert to their previous levels of happiness – unless they divorce, in which case their levels of happiness drop below the ones they had when they were single.

What's more, single people are not lonely and miserable – far from it. We tend to be less lonely than married people, because we are usually in more regular contact with friends, parents, neighbours and siblings than if we are in a couple.

Married people have The One, DePaulo says. Single people have The Ones.

I thought of all the friends and family I had . . . she was right, I had many Ones.

After all her research, DePaulo came to the conclusion that some people are just designed to be on their own – she calls these people 'single at heart'.

If you are single at heart, 'you are not single because you have "issues" or just haven't found a partner yet. Instead, living single is a way for you to lead your most meaningful and authentic life. Even people who are not single may be single at heart.'

Single-at-heart people tend to have a few things in common. They often value work, freedom and self-growth above romantic relationships. But the main characteristic of a single-at-heart person is how happy they are in their own company. While other people fear extended periods of time on their own, the single at heart revel in it.

She was describing me.

I loved work, had made a living out of self-growth (or navel-gazing, as my mum would put it), craved freedom and seemed to need more time alone than my friends did.

When I was a kid, I used to ask mum to tell the friends who phoned that I was in the bath because I didn't want to talk. As a teenager, when my friends feared missing out on the latest party, nine times out of ten I'd prefer to be reading or watching television. And in my twenties, as friends went off to music festivals, I stayed home. Being trapped with thousands of people for days was my idea of hell.

It wasn't that I felt anxious around crowds or that I didn't like people – I liked people a lot and on good days they liked me too – but after a few hours I'd always had enough.

It was only when I was in my thirties that I read Susan Cain's book *Quiet* and understood for the first time: I was an introvert. I recharged my batteries by being alone, while extroverts recharged by being together.

Maybe this was why Mum always said I would suit being a nun. 'You need a quiet life,' she'd say to me repeatedly. Sometimes I'd nod in agreement, and sometimes I felt angry with the sexless fate I was being handed.

Thing is: I didn't want to be a nun. I wanted to have fun, and love – but only when, and how, I wanted to. But could it work like that?

That afternoon, I went onto DePaulo's website and read every article she had written. With each one I felt that I understood myself in a way I had not before.

In one article she asks more questions to help you figure out if you are single at heart.

One asked: 'If you were in a committed relationship in the past, how did it feel?'

Like a trap. Like I stopped being me. Like I was going to suffocate. I thought of the last man I'd gone out with. A lovely, clever, kind man with not a single wrong thing except this: he wanted to do things together. All the time. He wanted to book holidays six months ahead. He wanted me to be a plus one to his friends' weddings. I hated it. I don't make plans! I wanted to scream: I might be dead in six months! I might not like you! You might not like me! No, no, no! But I didn't say that – instead I told myself I was wrong to feel like this and did my best to be a 'good girlfriend', until one day I couldn't do it any more.

De Paulo asks a follow-up question: 'If you tried romantic relationships in the past, how did you feel when they ended?'

I'd given the 'it's not you, it's me' speech in a pub on Tottenham Court Road. As soon as it was over I'd felt like I could breathe again.

DePaulo says this is common: 'People who are single at heart might feel relieved, even if the relationship wasn't bad at all. They just missed their single life. Something about being in a committed, coupled relationship felt constricting or just wrong. It wasn't who they really are.'

Oh my god, yes.

But then there was a question that made me think I might not be single at heart. DePaulo asks, when your friends and family members get married, how does that make you feel?

The article said that if you only feel sad because you'll be 'marginalized as your friend or family member enters the married club', that doesn't mean that you actually want to be married, just that you want your friends to stay available to you. However, if you look at people walking down the aisle and wish you had what they had, then single life may not be for you.

And that was the rub. Relationships made me feel suffocated and trapped, but when I went to weddings I felt the pain of not being loved or chosen. I knew that no man would stand in a suit, nervous and shuffling, holding a champagne glass up in a room full of round tables covered in white tablecloths and talk about the day he met me, and how he was so proud to call me his wife. I don't know how I knew this, but I did.

Was it because I knew deep down that the institution of the couple was not for me, or was it because I didn't think I deserved that love? It felt, in those moments, like the latter. I would sit with a pain in my chest, listening with a false smile to someone declaring love to my friend, and then go to the loo and cry because I would never be loved like that and I was missing out on one of the greatest parts of being alive.

So did that mean I was not, in fact, single at heart?

I put the kettle on to make more coffee. The radio was playing Frankie Goes to Hollywood, 'The Power of Love'. I wondered if I was fooling myself to think I was happy alone.

According to DePaulo, there *are* some downsides to being alone. First, you're not invited to couples-only dinner parties. I did not consider this to be a loss. Then there's the fact that governments and businesses favour couples, giving them tax breaks and preferential deals. I'd never thought of that. But the biggest issue for singles is the stigma we face.

DePaulo writes: 'If you are single, then you lose by definition. No matter what you can point to on your own behalf – spectacular accomplishments, a lifelong and caring convoy of relatives and friends, extraordinary altruism – none of it redeems you if you have no soulmate. Others will forever be scratching their heads and wondering what's wrong with you . . . It is like having a gymnastics routine lacking a key element that qualifies it for a perfect score; no matter how skilfully and gracefully you perform your routine, it will always be judged as lacking.'

Oh my god. That was so true. *So true.*

When the taxi driver made his comments about marriage, I wanted to tell him: 'Don't worry about me, mate! I've just written a book and travelled the world! I have the life I always dreamt of!'

But it would have been meaningless to him. The lady doth

protest too much – and anyway, who cares if you've written a book when you don't have a husband? DePaulo writes about how single people are put down at every turn. Do singles have close friends who are deeply important to them? Then they are described as 'just' friends. Do they have a sex life? Then they are sluts. No sex life? What a shame they aren't getting any. And singles devoted to their jobs? They are just compensating for not having a spouse. Are singles happy? They just think they are. Without a soulmate, they could never know true happiness.

All these messages make us think we must be fooling ourselves if we believe we are happy alone. They are why we go through the motions pretending to ourselves and others that we want to meet someone, even if our behaviour doesn't match our words.

DePaulo writes that single-at-heart people will say that they want to meet someone, when in reality 'doing what it would take to find that person seems to rank somewhere between deleting ancient emails from their inbox and cleaning out their sock drawer'. This summed it up exactly.

I had periods where I'd half-heartedly swipe on apps, but when it came down to it, I'd rather do anything but meet someone I didn't know in a pub on a Tuesday night. Dating felt like the tax I had to pay on being single. The thing I had to do. But maybe I didn't?

I watched the talk another three times, allowing the possibility to sink in: that it really was OK to be single. More than OK – it was the life that suited me, the life I'd been unconsciously choosing all along.

For so long, I'd taken for granted that to be single was a problem, a situation that needed fixing. I took it to mean that I was not wanted and not chosen. It never occurred to me that each time I had been chosen by someone, I walked away.

I teared up as DePaulo concluded her talk with these words: 'For way too long, we single people have been told that the only way we can be truly happy is to get married. Now we know that's just not so . . . single people, you know what to do: go out and live your single lives fully, joyfully and unapologetically.' Yes, Bella. I do! I mean, I will!

Just as I was embracing my singledom, my friend Daisy was crying over hers. She arrived at my front door with two wheelie suitcases after her relationship of six months ended. She had moved in with him after ten days together and now she was single and homeless, and dragging around a TK Maxx bag with what looked like a fleece dressing gown coming out of the top of it.

'I won't stay long,' she said.

'Stay as long as you like,' I replied.

'I'm sorry,' she said.

'What are you sorry for?'

'For this. For getting in your way.'

'You're not in my way.'

'It's for the best, isn't it?' she said, sitting on the sofa while I made us tea.

'Yes,' I said.

'I did the right thing?' she repeated.

'You did. You gave it a lot of chances.'

'Yeah . . .' She looked out of the window.

'And it wasn't right, what he did, was it?'

'Not at all. Really.'

'So I haven't made a mistake?'

'You haven't.'

I passed her tea.

'I've made a mess out of everything,' she said.

'You haven't,' I said.

'I'm thirty-five and alone again.'

'You're not alone, you're with me.'

'I've wasted so much time with the wrong men.'

Daisy and I had got to singlehood differently, but we were both there. As many of us were, it seemed.

Bella DePaulo had alerted me to the fact that a single-positivity movement was afoot, with several books written on the joy of being single.

The Unexpected Joy of Being Single by Catharine Gray was the most recent, then there was the critically acclaimed *All the Single Ladies* by Rebecca Traister, *Spinster* by Kate Bollick, *Singled Out* by Bella DePaulo and *Going Solo* by Eric Klinenberg.

'You should read this,' I told Daisy.

'What is it?' she asked.

I turned the book to face her.

'*The Unexpected Joy of Being Single*,' she read out loud.

'It's from the woman who wrote about the joy of being sober.'

'Oh yeah, I heard of that one.'

'This one is about how she was hooked on love and dating apps – and realized it was like booze, it was just a way to lose herself.'

'Hmmm,' she wasn't really listening but I kept going. I didn't see myself in Gray's behaviour, but I saw a lot of Daisy in it.

'Anyway, then she decided to stop dating for a year and she wrote two books, learned to drive and is saving up for a deposit to buy her own place. It's brilliant. She also says that it's just Hollywood bullshit that makes us feel like freaks for being single but actually over half of twenty-five- to forty-four-year-olds are single right now.'

Daisy looked at me.

'Is that true?'

'That's what it says.'

'But everyone I know is in a relationship.'

'Yeah, me too – well, no, not really. You're not and I'm not and Rachel isn't . . .'

Sometimes it can seem like everyone else is partnered when in fact they aren't.

Gray makes a compelling case for how society, films and songs have brainwashed us into thinking that coupledom is the meaning of life. The only way to be happy. Our one and only reason for living.

From the moment we're born, we're read fairy tales about the princess who lies in a coma until Prince Charming wakes her up, or poor Cinderella living a life of slavery until another Prince Charming invites her to the ball. As an adult, I knew that fairy tales weren't real, but as children our little subconscious minds soak these stories up.

And the stories kept coming. The endless magazine articles about how to bag the guy, ten ways to drive him wild in bed, the five things that will make him commit. Then the songs that played all day long; Mariah Carey singing, 'I can't live if living is without you'; LeAnn Rimes asking, 'How do I live without you? How do I breathe without you?'.

Never once did I think to say, LeAnn, I think you'll breathe just fine, and Mariah, you have more money than God and more power than most of the men around you – you will live an absolutely gorgeous life, whoever is in it. Even today, Beyonce's rallying cry to all the single ladies still has marriage as its end game.

'I'm going to do what she did – I'm going to go on a man ban,' Daisy said. 'I'm done with putting all my eggs into one dickhead.'

I felt pleased. Another convert to the single life.

After dinner we flicked through Netflix and decided to watch *He's Just Not That Into You*. I pressed play and settled into the sofa, looking forward to the safe and brightly coloured world of the romantic comedy. Escapist fluff that I'd been watching since I was a teenager. But this time the movie felt different.

It was shit. Not good shit. Just shit shit. Damaging shit, actually.

'Who acts like that?' I asked as Gigi, the main character, starts stalking a guy who is not calling her back. Daisy was on her phone and not listening.

'Nobody I know acts like that,' I repeated to Daisy. 'Stop it! Go home! Go home to your friends and your life,' I shouted at the screen.

I usually loved these cheesy movies, but until now I'd never ever thought about the toxic messages they gave me about what a single woman was: someone needy, unstable and irrational. Someone with bad hair, who spends hours staring at her phone, willing it to ring, while the men are off having a life.

Or there was the other kind of single woman – the damaged slut who has a heart of gold really, she just needs the right man to calm her down. Or the ruthless, hard career bitch who would at some point meet a child who would warm her cold, cold heart – and that child would be attached to a handsome, widowed father . . . How was I only just seeing this?

I closed my laptop.

'I can't watch this any more, it's insulting. I mean, even Bridget Jones—' I started. 'Even Bridget Jones – I mean, I love her, but she's telling us that all single women sit around in their pyjamas, drinking wine and crying at weddings. But maybe being a single woman doesn't have to be anything like that? Maybe,' I said, sitting up and warming to my theme, 'maybe we've all embodied the Bridget Jones clichés because that was the only part on offer! There haven't been any scripts with "happy single woman has a great life without getting married". But maybe we can write a new script!'

Daisy's phone beeped. She looked down and smiled.

'Who are you texting?'

'A guy I went to school with.'

I didn't say anything.

'He's just separated.'

I raised my eyebrows.

'I know, but he's an INFJ and a Leo, which is good for me.'

'How do you know his personality type?'

'He just did a test online.'

'When?'

'Just now, when we were watching the film.'

'Did you ask him to?'

'Yeah.'

'And he did it?'

'Yes.'

I went to bed, tutting every time I heard giggling and the pinging of messages. I flicked through my phone. No messages.

'Can you put your phone on silent?' I called to Daisy as her phone beeped again. I worried I was slipping into another single stereotype: the miserable spinster.

Except spinsters weren't always miserable. The next day I went to the hairdresser to get my greys done. Under the heat, I read in Gray's book that in the Middle Ages the term 'spinster' didn't have the negative connotations that it does today. In fact, 'spinsters' were women who had an independent income from spinning yarn, and so they did not have to marry; they could if they chose to, but many chose not to. They were the female equivalent of a bachelor. 'Spinster' only became a slur when settlers went to America and needed to build up the population – then single women without children were demonized for not helping the cause. They were accused of being witches and bullied into getting married in order to provide a better income for their families. And the reality was that for most women, marriage was a financial necessity.

And this was the case until very recently.

Gray shares some shocking stats. Irish women couldn't buy a house outright, without a male co-signee, until 1976. Women couldn't open a bank account in their own name until 1975 in the UK, nor apply for a loan or a credit card without their father's signature and permission, until the mid seventies.

In short, until the late seventies the vast number of women in the UK and Ireland needed a husband in order to secure a roof over their heads. The independence we now have is a very new thing.

As Gray concludes: 'Being single is a supremely modern privilege women can now enjoy without being driven to join a nunnery.'

I was so lucky to be living in the time I was.

As I walked out of the hairdressers with the kind of swagger you only get from good hair, I realized that mum was right. I had a freedom that previous generations could only dream of.

How ridiculous not to enjoy all that. How ungrateful, actually. Women had fought and died to create a society that allowed women like me to live exactly as we wanted. And around the world, so many still couldn't live freely. I was part of a new generation of women who didn't have to be dependent on anyone – economically, socially or sexually. Seen this way, maybe my single status was not a failure but an evolution. And also a huge privilege.

It was time to stop second-guessing my freedom and start to celebrate it.

But how?

Some women were going as far as marrying themselves. White dresses, rings, the lot. It was called sologamy. I knew this because Facebook had alerted me to a talk in Camden by women who had said 'I do' to themselves.

I couldn't believe the coincidence of the event coming up on my Facebook feed when I was looking at single positivity, but then I realized that my phone was listening to my conversations. (You see, we're never really alone, are we?)

I went with Rachel and Daisy.

There were twelve of us in the audience, in office tights and damp shoes, our chairs pointing towards two women who had married themselves.

I crossed my legs and my arms and got ready for a good session of eye-rolling, but it was actually quite good. One woman talked about how she'd had enough of toxic relationships and hating herself. On her fiftieth birthday she and her best friend had a tiny ceremony in a church. She got a ring, made vows to love herself and to stop looking for someone to complete her. They threw confetti and ate cake. She said it was one of the most tender experiences of her life.

'Well, I married myself on the rebound!' said the next woman. I suspected this was a line she used often.

She talked about how she'd had a bad break-up and a parent had died. She realized that she'd spent her life twisting herself into a role that was never for her, in an attempt to tick the required boxes. So she decided to skip the boxes and buy herself a ring.

Rachel leant towards me. 'Is this just an excuse to buy yourself a ring?'

The discussion opened up to the audience. We talked about how when you're single, you are forever celebrating other people's milestones, other people's engagements, weddings, births, yet there are no celebrations for us. We talked about the feeling of being defined by your relationship status – down to the whole 'Miss' and 'Mrs' thing. A woman with bright-red lipstick, who described herself as a therapist and an Uber driver, talked about how she asked to be referred to as 'Ms' in correspondence, but her solicitor refused to use it. So she started sending him letters that addressed him as 'Mrs'. He didn't like it.

Two hours later, we walked out into the rain and chicken shops of Camden High Street. 'That wasn't as mad as I thought it would be,' said Rachel, as we stood on the pavement.

'If I had the money, I'd throw myself a wedding,' said Daisy.

'Would you?' I asked, horrified.

'Who doesn't want to be the centre of attention for the day? And wear a nice dress?' she asked.

'Not me,' I said. I'd never dreamt of the big white dress . . . but it wasn't true to say I'd never thought of getting married. When I was younger, I pictured being in a register office in a trouser suit. Probably because that was what my mum had done.

'What about you? Are you going to buy yourself a ring?' I asked Rachel. She looked down at her hands. She was already wearing four.

The event had inspired me, but Rachel wasn't convinced.

Later, Rachel and I went to get a drink. Daisy had gone off to meet her INF-whatever. 'I get the whole "you don't need anyone to complete you" thing, but it makes me feel like I'm being un-feminist for *wanting* someone,' she said. 'I don't want a partner because I think I'm nothing without a man, I just like being in a couple. I like cooking dinner and going on holiday together . . .'

'I hate the "what's for dinner?" chat,' I said.

'So are you saying you don't want a relationship with anyone? That you're going to be single for the rest of your life?' she asked.

'Yeah, maybe.'

'And you'd be OK with that?'

'Yeah, I really think I would.'

'You don't think you're running away?'

'From what?' I asked.

'Intimacy. Being vulnerable. Getting hurt.'

I shrugged. I didn't know. Why were single people always accused of running away? Couldn't you say that couples were running away from being alone?

Rachel told me about her latest dates. A guy who talked about himself all night only to text her later asking how many dates they'd need to go on before they went on holiday together. Another guy she'd had a great first date with, but who'd cancelled their second, saying he was sick, and then blocked her.

'If you're a woman over thirty-five looking for children you are the opposite of catnip – you literally repel men. And I don't blame them – I'd want someone younger and easier than me,' she said. 'Are you sure you don't want kids?' she asked me.

'I'm not sure of anything,' I said.

Almost every woman in my life seemed to know from their late twenties that they wanted kids. Gemma, my best friend in Ireland; Sarah, my work friend who had just moved out to the suburbs. Pretty much everyone I went to school with. If it didn't happen naturally, they spent tens of thousands on IVF to make it happen.

'Did you always want them?' I asked.

'Yes.'

'But why do you want them?'

'I don't know. I just do. It's just what I've always pictured for myself . . .'

'I don't picture that.'

'You're lucky.'

'Maybe – or maybe I'll wake up at sixty and realize I've missed the point of life.'

She shrugged.

'If you don't want a boyfriend or children, then fuck it – enjoy your life, take a lover!'

I scrunched up my face. 'I'm too repressed to take a lover,' I said.

'Well, get unrepressed,' Rachel said, with the same straightforwardness she applied to her own life.

On the train I thought about what I'd have to do to become unrepressed and take a lover. The idea made me feel liberated and sexy and . . . not me. But I'd like to be that person.

Just because I was ambivalent about relationships didn't mean I wanted to be celibate. I didn't, but I had hang-ups around sex. I was a forty-year-old Catholic schoolgirl, and not the fun, naughty kind – the 'everything is a sin' kind. I was pretty much living out my mum's premonition that I'd make a good nun. And I didn't want to keep living like that.

I wanted beautiful sex. Transcendent, earth-moving sex.

I also wanted to be, well, good at it.

As someone who had spent most of their adult life single, I always worried I was shit in bed. Everyone else – all the 'normal' people – had years of practice and knew what they were doing. I didn't. When it came to sex, I was still an awkward teenager. It was my secret shame.

I wanted to get over that shame, to become a woman of the world, a master lover. I wanted to have sexy underwear that actually got worn in sexy situations.

The train was full of tipsy young couples sitting close, heads on shoulders, holding hands. I smiled. As I looked at them, I imagined a whole life mapped out for them. Of messy dates, moving in together, getting married . . .

In a couple, there is a path in front of you.

As a single woman, not dating, there isn't a path. Or at least not one that I'd want to go down.

I'd have to make up my own.

But what would it look like? What does a full, happy, sexual life look like for a single woman? What did it look like for me in my forties? A life full of love and freedom?

It might sound like an old-fashioned question to ask in the twenty-first century, but the truth was I didn't see any women living that life. What I saw were people who were either single or not. And those who were single were trying not to be.

I knew from my year of self-help that relationships were the single most important factor in a happy life. Study after study showed that it was the people in our lives, not money, status or possessions, that made us happy – but surely that didn't have to be romantic relationships?

In *Singled Out*, Bella DePaulo had written about how the obsession with the couple and the nuclear family is the 'narrowest construal of intimacy' that has ever existed. She writes that for most of human history 'the tendrils of love and affection reached out to family, friends, and community, reached back to ancestors, and reached up to the heavens' – they were never meant to focus on just one person.

What if I put my tendrils of love and affection out into the world, rather than just on dating apps? Instead of putting all my energy into finding The One, could I nurture relationships with The Ones? Could I learn how to be a better friend, daughter and sister? Could I get over my sexual inhibitions enough to have lovers? But how would I even find lovers? Would I have to go on hook-up apps?

When I got home, I put the heating on, lit a candle and poured a glass of wine.

At the sologamy event they had talked about writing vows to oneself. I opened my journal and wrote VOWS at the top.

I vow to live my life fully. Now. As it is.
I vow to love myself as I am and to not think I'm a weirdo for
  being single.
I vow not to see myself as a lesser person because I'm not
  married and don't have children.
I vow to see my singleness as an opportunity, not an affliction.
I vow to find love in ways that suit me. Whatever they
  might be.
I vow to stop running away and being scared of sex and men.
I vow to treasure my friendships and to do more to sustain
  them.

I wondered if I should buy myself a ring, but I decided my first act of self-love would be to take fiscal responsibility.

I also thought about buying a fabulous jumpsuit which I'd wear with giant hoop earrings and red lipstick. That's how I pictured an empowered single woman in her forties: with red lips and wearing a jumpsuit, or a trouser suit. But this wasn't about how I looked. It was about the life I wanted to lead.

A mission formulated:

I would find a way to have great sex outside of a traditional relationship. I'd become a better friend, daughter, sister, and maybe even do some community work. I would explore love in its many forms. I'd read books, go to workshops and find out what happens when the story doesn't end with marriage and children.

I would find a new happy ever after.

As I lay in bed smiling, I could hear Daisy letting herself in. I felt a pang of envy at her date, and tried to push aside the fear that I was, as Rachel suggested, running away.

2

Self-Love

'If you're staying single, you need to get some self-love going,' Daisy said, over breakfast.

'Yes, I was thinking that too,' I said.

At the sologomy event they'd talked about how marrying yourself meant roasting yourself a whole chicken if you fancied it and eating it at a table with a tablecloth and a candle. It meant realizing that you are whole and good right now, and that you don't need someone else to validate you. You deserve the fancy china . . .

I didn't have any fancy china. Maybe it was time to buy some? Roast a chicken?

In my self-help mission I had read a book called *You Can Heal Your Life* by Louise Hay, which told me to stand in front of the mirror while repeating the words: 'I love and approve of myself, I love and approve of myself.'

It was the last book I'd read and by the time I'd got to it I'd had enough of looking in the metaphorical mirror. I'd skipped through the exercises that were designed to help me love myself.

I could try it again, I supposed.

But Daisy wasn't talking about that kind of self-love.

'I mean self-pleasure,' she said. 'If you want great sex, it starts with yourself,' she said.

I felt my cheeks heat up. I scraped butter on my toast.

'Have you watched Layla Martin?'

'No.'

'She's great – she's got loads of videos on YouTube. She's the one who got me into all the tantra stuff.'

I had never asked Daisy for details when she referred to her 'tantra stuff'. I imagined a mound of oiled-up bodies writhing like sexy worms, and it scared the shit out of me.

'This jam is really nice,' I said, with a mouth full of toast.

'She has a great jade-egg course that she runs online. If you order the egg through her you get access to online tutorials.'

'What? No! I don't want to stick a stone inside me.'

'Fair enough, love. You don't need to. There are books you can read. *Pussy: A Reclamation*, *Love Your Lady Landscape* . . .'

'*Love Your Lady Landscape*?' I practically spat out the words.

'Yeah. It's great, but I'd probably read *Pussy* first. It says you should wake up every morning and look at your pussy in the mirror and say, "Good morning, gorgeous!" And she reckons it'll change your life. It helps you fall in love with yourself.'

'What? You looked at your—' I couldn't say 'pussy'. 'You looked at your vagina in the mirror every morning and talked to it?' How was she acting like this was normal?

'Actually, the vagina is just the inside bit. Your outside bits are called the vulva, but in the book she prefers the term "pussy".'

Daisy must have seen a look of horror on my face because she stopped talking and got up from the table as I sat eating my toast like a prude. Was I a prude? Maybe I was, but how did she think it was OK to talk about masturbation at 8 a.m.?

I did not talk about masturbation with anyone. Not over breakfast, not over anything. Even the word made me feel ashamed. Not that I didn't do it – I did. But it was a private, often furtive affair that usually made me feel a bit ashamed afterwards.

But I felt ashamed of my shame. I was out of touch. Literally.

Masturbation was mainstream now. Boots and Superdrug were selling vibrators. The BBC had done a news item about how good it was for women's health. Millennials swapped notes on podcasts about their favourite vibrators in the same way they'd swap notes on mascara. A vagina museum had opened in Camden, and artists were posting whimsical illustrations of vaginas – or vulvas, I should say – on Instagram. 'Put it away!' I wanted to shout.

As Daisy got ready to leave the flat she turned back to me and said, 'Love, I hope you don't mind me saying this . . . but you do have some hang ups around this stuff.'

She was right, I did have hang ups. Around my body, my sexuality and my . . . whatever we're calling it. And if I had learned anything from my year of self-help experiments, it was that the less I wanted to do something, the more I probably needed to do it.

I googled jade eggs and clicked on links that took me to stories about Goop being fined $140,000 for making unsubstantiated claims about what they could do. Gwyneth was still selling them, with the promise that they 'harness the power of energy work, crystal healing and a Kegel-like physical practice.' Whatever that meant.

She called them 'yoni' eggs. I googled 'yoni' and discovered that it was spiritual speak for pussy, which was girly speak for vagina, which was often inaccurately used to describe the vulva. This was a minefield.

I clicked through a few articles. Most featured gynaecologist Jen Gunter, who was advising women to stay away from the eggs, warning that they could give you toxic shock syndrome.

That phrase brought back memories of reading *More* magazine in my sixth-form common room. There were always articles about toxic shock brought on by leaving your tampon in too long. It turned out to be much less of a thing than we'd been led to believe . . . as were the articles about how to dress from 'day to night'. All these funny messages we got from the age of thirteen about what being a woman was – potentially fatal, and having to dress perfectly for every occasion.

Dr Gunter also warned that we should avoid putting parsley up there, and garlic too. And that we shouldn't steam our fannies, or we could end up with third-degree burns. Were people actually doing this?

It was all mad.

I took a shower.

When I got back to my desk, I looked up *Pussy: A Reclamation*, just to further prove to myself that this was all stupid and I wanted no part of it.

'Get ready to encounter a book that will change your experience as a woman,' the Amazon blurb told me, before saying that it would teach me 'the key practices required to seek and speak your deepest truth, no matter what.' Well, that sounded good. I was shit at speaking my deepest truth. The blurb went on: *How to end the war with your body.* Well, if she could do that then surely she should be given the Nobel peace prize? *How to trade overwork and resentment for gratitude-filled, passionate contributions.* If she could rid me of overwork and resentment, I didn't know who I'd be, but I'd like to find out. *Why a woman's sensual awareness is critical for her spiritual, intellectual and emotional health.* I didn't have any sensual awareness.

As I read, I felt that familiar combination of wanting to roll my eyes at the cheesiness of it all, while hoping deep down that this book would offer *the* answer. To what I didn't know. Sexual liberation? Unfettered self-confidence? Untold wealth that would shower down on me while I looked lavishly sexy? Men falling at my feet?

And then I read the final promise: '*Pussy* delivers the tools and practices a woman requires to do and be whatever she wants in this life. It's a call for her to tune in, turn on, and not drop out – but live more richly, fully and lusciously than she ever thought she could.'

That was exactly what I was looking for. A rich, full, luscious life. One in which I could do and be whatever I wanted. I didn't know what 'tune in, turn on, and not drop out' involved, but I was willing to find out. I was also relieved that none of the blurb seemed to be about masturbation.

I ordered the book.

'*Pussy*.' (It begins.) The word made me wince. 'It's arguably the most powerful pejorative word in the English language.'

Was it, though? I mean, I didn't love it but . . . was it that bad? Surely the c– word was worse?

No, says the book's author, Regena Thomashauer: if you call a man a pussy, you're insulting his manhood. Say it to a woman and you're objectifying her.

Say the word out loud, she suggests.

My throat tightened up. I didn't want to say it. I felt an itch at the back of my throat. I wanted to stay quiet.

'Pussy,' I whispered, sitting at my desk.

Thomashauer reckons that when women say it, they smile. She urges readers to reclaim the word, to reclaim our power.

It didn't make me smile. But I couldn't find any word that didn't make me wince. 'Cunt' sounded powerful, but I didn't have the guts to use a term that's considered one of the most offensive terms in the world. But why was it so offensive? Why was the word describing the place where all life begins considered the worst insult you could throw at someone?

'Vulva', on the other hand, sounded prissy. 'Vagina' sounded medical, and apparently only describes the inside bits.

Thomashauer says that the majority of women were raised to either give their genitals silly names such 'kitty', 'cuckoo', 'little princess' and, weirdest of all, 'purse' – purse! – or they say vagina when they are actually referring to the vulva. But most common of all, they were taught to call it nothing at all. 'When we have no common language to describe that which is most essentially feminine about us, we have no way to locate our power as a woman,' she writes.

When we have no word for something, the implication is that it's so shameful it can't even be talked about.

This shame pervades every area of our life, according to Thomashauer, and is part of the reason women continue to be plagued with self-doubt and self-loathing. It's why girls don't put their hands up in class. Why women get paid less than men. Why even the most successful female business-women say they feel like frauds.

This seemed like a lot to put on a pussy.

But as I read on, it was hard to completely disagree with her case.

In one of the opening sections, Thomashauer asks us how we feel about being a woman. What were we taught about being a woman from our family? Our culture? Our religion? Is being a woman exciting? Discouraging? Neutral? On a scale of one to ten, how much do you enjoy being a woman?

I'd never thought about any of this before.

I got my journal out. Floral. Paperchase. I don't know why I bought it. It was too girly. I turned the pages, past the vows I'd written to myself after the sologamy event. I put the word *pussy* at the top of the page and wrote out the first question: Was it exciting to become a woman?

What a stupid question. Of course not: it involved boobs and periods and being told not to talk to strange men. In short: bodily fluids and fear.

I wrote out the second question: How do you feel about being a woman?

Another stupid question. What was the point of this?

I got up and went to the loo. Then I put the kettle on, opened the fridge, closed it and opened it again. I wondered if I was hungry, but I'd just had lunch. I made a cup of tea and sat down again.

How do I feel about being a woman?

I wondered if I had any chocolate. I got up to look in the cupboards. I didn't. I sat down again.

How do I feel about being a woman?

I felt impatient. Get over yourself, don't make a fuss. Don't talk about being a woman because it's . . . it's . . . nothing. Being a woman was nothing. So I wrote that down.

Being a woman is nothing. It's— my pen hovered. *It's less than a man. I don't enjoy it but I don't dislike it either – it's nothing. A bit embarrassing. Nothing to celebrate. It feels a bit like it's embarrassing to be a woman . . . like something I don't want to talk about. Not awful either, as I am a straight, white, able-bodied woman living in a Western country.*

I had written the word 'nothing' three times, and the word 'embarrassing' twice.

I drank my tea and looked out the window and saw a young woman in white jeans and a short puffa. I did not have the figure to wear an outfit like that. I envied her.

I picked up my pen again.

Being a woman means never quite living up to the mark. It means never being attractive enough or young enough.

And then I found myself writing: *Being a woman means being scared of attack.*

I moved on to the next question: What did I think my job was as a woman?

Well, that was easy. I wrote quickly: *Be pretty and nice and quiet and good and help others and be agreeable. And if you aren't pretty enough then you have to double up in all the other areas to compensate.*

Next: What did I think of the word 'feminine'?

It made me cringe, and think of pink bedrooms, perfume, fakeness, Barbies and . . . feminine hygiene products.

Then: What did my religion tell me about being a woman?

Again, easy. *Women ruined everything!*

I remembered Sister Mary Loretto telling us about Adam and Eve at school. This lovely naked couple lived happily in paradise until Eve ate the apple she was not meant to eat. I remember going home distraught. 'Why did she do it?' I asked mum. 'If she didn't eat the apple we would all be in the Garden of Eden now! Life would be heaven if it wasn't for her!' I believed it completely and was furious with Eve for messing everything up.

I have no memory of what mum said back, or whether she mounted a defence on behalf of the first woman. Probably not. She had sausages to cook and clothes to wash.

So it was just as well I also learned about the Virgin Mary, who was quiet and pretty and nice and did what was asked of her, including having a baby without having sex . . . I could emulate her. Also, in all my school books Mary wore blue, which was my favourite colour.

I was aware of Mary Magdalene also being part of the

picture, but she seemed grown-up in ways my child's mind couldn't understand.

Speaking of God: Thomashauer suggests we say out loud the words God and Goddess to see how they feel.

'God,' I said out loud at my desk. It felt strong. True. Powerful.

'Goddess,' I said, and grimaced. 'Goddess' was pretend, stupid, girly, weak, a fantasy.

By the time I'd closed my journal, the penny had dropped: I didn't like being a woman. I was . . . a misogynist.

That night, I lay in bed listening to Daisy's phone pinging. Things were moving fast with the INF-whatever. I worried for her but didn't want to be a downer. She had her life to live and I had mine.

My life to live as a woman.

Something I did not like being, which was news to me.

The book explained that we live in a patriarchal society that celebrates the masculine and devalues the feminine, which is why so many women hate themselves.

It wasn't always this way.

There was a time when women were worshipped and powerful, considered to be the source of all life. In ancient Egypt, when the crops were planted, women would stand along the field and raise their skirts and flash at the field of wheat. They would say, 'Wheat, may you grow as high as my pussy.' In Ireland, women would flash at the sea to ensure their fisherman husbands had a calm voyage, such was their power. There were hundreds of twelfth-century carvings of naked women with huge vulvas outside churches, of all places. These are called sheela na gigs, and the images are thought to represent fertility and life, and to ward against evil spirits. Historically, when death was everywhere, women did something exceptional: they created life.

I was amazed to read that women had ever been revered this way, and sad that I'd never heard any of this history before, even in my all-girls school. The fact that I was so shocked that women were ever respected – worshipped, even – made me feel sadder still. How far we had fallen.

Fortunately, Regena had the answer: pussy rehab.

Seriously.

Pussy rehab.

Oh, Reg.

As Daisy had told me, Thomashauer recommends starting each morning by looking in the mirror at your pussy and saying, 'Good morning, beautiful.' She says that when we do this, men smile at you and meetings go well. Next she suggests that we set an alarm, and that every hour we touch our pussy and check in with her. She says our pussy will feel soothed by the attention. Finally, if you have any particular dilemmas, why not touch your pussy or look at her in the mirror and ask her for the answers? Like a hairy magic eight ball. You can ask questions such as, 'Pussy, do you want me to wear the red dress or the blue?' Or, 'Pussy, do you want to go out tonight or stay in?' You can also consult your GPS – Giant Pussy in the Sky – about where to park.

And if that wasn't nuts enough, Thomashauer says that some of her pupils like to get a pussy puppet to talk to. A. Pussy. Puppet.

This was straight-up madness, the kind of thing that gave women a bad name. And yet this book was making me think about things I had never thought about before. For every ridiculous passage there was a story of female empowerment that had me sitting up straight, scribbling exclamation marks in the margins.

I put my hand between my legs over my pyjamas. It felt warm and twisty and nervous down there.

'Pussy,' I said. Silently. 'Should I do all this crazy stuff?'

A strong *yes* came from inside me.

I was shocked: first to know that my pussy could talk and secondly that it wanted anything to do with this craziness.

My head, however, thought differently. It said a firm *no* to looking in a mirror and talking to my pussy. That *no* was like a brick wall.

'How is it meant to change your life?' my sister asked, as we walked towards the park. A car alarm was going off.

'Something to do with owning your feminine power and . . . falling in love with yourself. I dunno.'

I had spent five days not looking at my pussy and it was bothering me. Why was it such a big deal?

'Don't you think it's weird that we don't look at this really important part of our body?' I asked.

'No. It's tucked away. Why would you look at it? I don't look at the soles of my feet.'

'Yeah, but I don't feel disgusted by the thought of the soles of my feet.'

'I do,' she said.

'What did we call it when we were growing up?' I asked.

'Fanny,' she said. 'Or front bottom?'

I laughed.

'But seriously, what's this got to do with being happy single?'

'I think it's about loving yourself as a woman, whether you're single or not. And loving your body . . .'

We kept walking.

We saw two little ones standing in a giant puddle and jumping up and down. I stopped and smiled.

'Are you getting broody?' Sheila asked.

'No,' I said. Irritated by the question.

'OK,' said Sheila, 'I'd better head back, I've got boxing. Have fun falling in love with yourself. Make sure you don't get notions . . .'

Getting notions was an Irish phrase for getting ahead of yourself. Getting too big for your boots. It was said jokingly but the message was deadly serious. You should never, ever like yourself too much. If you did, you could be sure that someone would slap you down.

It made me mad. This idea that liking yourself was a sin.

Fuck. That.

I marched home and took the mirror from my bathroom.

It needed a clean, so I sprayed it and got distracted squeezing blackheads. Then I remembered that I was supposed to be examining my feminine magnificence, not picking holes in myself.

I got angry again. This is what we do as women, isn't it? Look in the mirror and find flaws. We don't look in the mirror to see ourselves, we look in the mirror to attack ourselves.

No more. Enough.

I got on my bed and took off my jeans and knickers.

I positioned the mirror between my legs, but it fell over. I got a pillow and propped it up . . . and got a flash of – oh, God, it was on the magnification side. No, no, no.

I flipped it over to the normal side.

Thomashauer writes: 'You will see a lush landscape reveal itself . . . Her colour can include palest peach, the rosiest coral, the deepest red . . . You may gasp and fail to find the words, like trying to describe a sunset on the phone.'

I looked down at the mirror propped against my pillow.

My pussy did not look like a sunset.

Instead it was a mush of flaps and folds, and some white hairs. This was depressing. The first time I went looking for the source of my power, I already had white hair.

Thomashauer says there are five stages to pussy rehab. First, there is revulsion. Then there is a scientific detachment. Stage three is when you become an affectionate researcher. By stage four you are a 'pussy aficionado' who takes 'great pride in her landscape, her architecture, the potential that comes with owning clitoral pleasure.' Finally, the final stage of pussy mastery is 'rapture'. At this point 'we weep tears of gratitude and astonishment at the privilege of being a woman. We hear Handel's Hallelujah Chorus.'

I was a long way from singing choirs. Instead, I could hear more Phil Collins coming from Michael's flat downstairs and a drill digging up the road.

Phil Collins and a drill.

I pulled up my knickers and jeans and jumped out of bed, pretending that none of that had happened.

That night I dreamt my labia were hanging down by my knees.

I called Sarah and asked her if she'd ever looked.

'Not since having kids. I remember doing it when I read *Are You There God? It's Me, Margaret*. But then I got freaked out when I did it again in my twenties and I looked completely different, the flaps were way bigger and it looked like a badly packed kebab.'

I laughed.

'Do you really want to do all this again?' Sarah asked.

'What?'

'All the self-help stuff. I thought you'd decided you were done trying to fix yourself?'

'I'm not trying to fix stuff, I just want to learn more about things, and relationships. What's wrong with that?'

'Nothing, just go easy on yourself,' she said. 'Look, I have to go, there's someone at the door.'

Daisy had started looking again, and seemed to find it a perfectly normal thing to do. I didn't understand how she had no reaction to it and I was having such a huge one.

'Do you want to do a vagina timeline?' she asked me.

'What?'

'It's where you write down everything that's happened or everything you've felt around your vagina, like from the first time you looked at it, or was told its name, to your first sexual touch. It's very healing.'

Another brick wall.

'No!' I snapped. *No, no, no.* Why did she keep saying this stuff? How was she so OK with it all?

'Did you know that the clitoris is the only part of the body that doesn't age?' she asked.

I told her I had to go see my mum.

On the walk I felt confused and upset. Why was this bothering me so much? Why hadn't I looked at this part of my body before? Why, when I looked at it, did it make me feel so sad? And wrong and ugly?

I didn't tell mum about looking at my own pussy. Instead I asked her if she loved herself.

'No,' she replied.

'Why not?'

'I don't know.'

'Do you like yourself?'

'Not really.'

'That's terrible,' I said.

'Well, I don't hate myself.'

'Why don't you like yourself?'

'I wasn't brought up to like myself.'

We watched *The Voice*. A woman got booted off. 'I just wanted to show my children that if you've got a talent, you've got to share your gift with the world,' she said to will.i.am.

'Shame nobody wants your gift,' said mum to the TV.

Thomashauer writes: 'If I learn self-hatred and self-doubt from my mother then I must adapt to her point of view if I want to show my love to her. Otherwise I'll be disrespecting her. I must hate myself because I love her and I want her to love me.'

Thomashauer says that women are brought up to serve everyone but themselves. They are taught to offer their bodies for other people's pleasure. Cook meals for other people's enjoyment. They give give give until they have nothing left and then they wonder why they are burnt out.

In many ways I did not see myself in this. As a single woman with no children, I was not giving myself to others the way my friends were. And I certainly wasn't cooking meals for anyone's enjoyment. Not even my own. And yet, in other ways I saw this pattern of always being nice, always offering myself up, always saying sure, I had time to talk, even when I was tired. Offering to meet people near them, if that was easier. 'No problem!' was probably the most-used phrase, along with, 'I'm easy!'.

Easy. Resentful, more like.

Thomashauer says that to reclaim their lives, women must reclaim pleasure – for themselves. She advocates buying yourself flowers, wining and dining yourself, rubbing beautiful creams into your skin and looking in the mirror to admire yourself. She recommends throwing out everything in your wardrobe that doesn't make you feel radiant. Looking after your appearance is not vanity, it's a 'sacred duty'. Then you can lie on the bed and stroke yourself all over, treating yourself like a precious lover.

The idea of all this made me want to be sick in my mouth.

But I did it. Except for the throwing out non-radiant clothes bit. If I did that I'd have had nothing to wear.

Daisy was out again, and so I embarked on an evening of romancing myself. I didn't have a bath in my flat, so I took a shower and rubbed cream into my body afterwards. I noticed how brusque and impatient I was as I did it. Trying to get it over with.

Then I stood in front of the mirror and looked at my body for the first time in a long time.

After years spent flagellating myself for not looking good enough, I had developed a more enlightened approach: I no longer criticized my body, I ignored it.

While this was liberating in a way, it was also sad. It wasn't self-love, it was self-negation.

But now I looked. Really looked.

I was greeted with the body of a middle-aged woman who was not getting away with her cheese-on-toast habit quite as much as she liked to think. Straight away I homed in on the parts that had got bigger, wobblier and fuller since I'd last looked. My boobs were sagging and my waist broader. I now had back fat too, which was depressing.

I didn't want to be this Bridget Jones cliché worrying about the size of her arse, but I was and I hated that. Thanks to body positivity I didn't just feel bad about my arse, I now felt bad about feeling bad about it. Like I was letting the side down.

I was supposed to love myself as I was. Embrace my curves. Celebrate my cellulite.

But I couldn't.

Thomashauer says that she had never considered herself to be beautiful, but she trained herself to by looking in the mirror and practising picking out the bits she loved.

So I tried to see the positives – my full hair, my curves, my nice boobs . . . but it was like a box ticking exercise. My heart wasn't in it.

I saw white hairs sprouting from my chin.

Wrinkles in the corner of my eyes.

I had thoughts about how nobody could fancy a body like this.

I put my towel back on and opened some wine.

Still in my towel, I chopped up bright red peppers and put them in the oven to roast with some onions.

While the vegetables were cooking, I was going to get into my pyjamas, but I stopped myself. The whole point was to dress up and feel good. I took the underwear I'd bought for the Greek out of its paper. Should I put it on? It felt ridiculous to put sexy underwear on to eat roast peppers alone . . . but then it also felt stupid keeping them hostage in white paper. I put them on under a silk dressing gown I had bought myself as a birthday present. The silk felt like a cool caress on my skin.

The experience of eating alone, in my fancy knickers and silk dressing gown at a candlelit table, felt surprisingly tender. I was almost shy of myself. But soon a voice popped into my head telling me that this was stupid and tragic, and that I had to resort to romancing myself because nobody else would.

The voice told me that if I kept eating pasta nobody would want to romance me.

I finished dinner and took myself to bed where I was supposed to stroke myself as I would a precious lover. As I started to stroke my legs, my head fought it. This was ridiculous. Pathetic. Tragic. I would not allow myself to believe that my body was beautiful – it wasn't. It was flawed and fat and hairy . . . and I did not deserve to be touched like I was something precious. I wasn't. And anyway, this sensuality wasn't good, it was conceited and wrong. Morally wrong.

I tried to talk myself around. How could it be wrong? It was just me in my bed. I wasn't hurting anyone . . . but still, it actually felt wrong to love myself in this way. In any way.

For years, Thomashauer was sexually shut down, frozen in shame, self-doubt and inadequacy. Then she became 'cliterate', discovering the limitless pleasures that could come from the clitoris, which is the only part of the human body whose only known function is pleasure. Why had I never heard this before? But of course, I hadn't. The nuns weren't big on chat about female pleasure – but I couldn't just blame it on Catholicism. The full size and shape of the clitoris was only mapped in the 1990s. Then it was discovered that the clitoris isn't just a little dot – hence all the jokes about men not being able to find it – but is in fact a wishbone shape that runs inside the body alongside the vagina.

Thomashauer says that we should take the existence of the clitoris as a sign that women are built for pleasure. Literally. It's our fuel, our make-up – even though society tells us the exact opposite.

She says that most women spend their lives waiting like Sleeping Beauty for Prince Charming without realizing that they have all they need to turn themselves on. Her life changed when she started to become her own lover.

Self-pleasure did more for her than years of therapy and self-help. It filled her body with feel-good chemicals and gave her a rush of energy and confidence. She became the woman she knew she was meant to be.

Thomashauer describes her orgasm thus: 'I felt like a butterfly, stung like a bee, soared like a shooting star, flowed like a river, poured with thick, gooey, oozing, honey-textured streams of sensation . . . Felt both the eternity and ephemeral nature of being human.'

My own sexual exploration went thus: a quick, functional wank, come quickly and a dirty 'let's pretend that didn't happen' feeling. I didn't make love to myself – I treated myself like a drunken one night stand I'd be embarrassed about the next day.

For the next few weeks I tried, and failed, to prioritize pleasure.

The book suggests taking regular dance breaks to flood our bodies with happy chemicals and to celebrate our sexiness. I loved jumping up and down to some house track and regularly went to something called ecstatic dance sessions – kind of sober raves – but when it came to dancing sexily, I felt clunky and inhibited. I couldn't do it – shake my hips, enjoy the feeling of my body, dare to think that I might be sexy. I just couldn't. It felt big-headed and ridiculous. I was not sexy. More than that, it felt dangerous in some way. Even though I was alone in my kitchen, I felt like dancing sexily was provocative and looking for trouble.

Being a woman means being scared of attack.

As soon as I felt pleasure, I put the brakes on. Not just sexual pleasure, but any pleasure. It felt decadent and selfish and lazy . . . get back to work, I told myself. Call your mother.

Be a good girl. Stay safe. Who do you think you are? A host of messages came into my head when I dared to relax and maybe think that everything was good and I was good . . .

Thomashauer suggests something called 'Pant-Free Friday' to add a frisson to your week. It does what it says on the tin – you go without underwear on a Friday. In fairness, this was something I often did when I'd run out of clean knickers, but this time I did it in the hope it would make me feel sexy. It didn't. My jeans were too tight and rubbed me. I walked home from the greengrocers like John Wayne.

Against my better judgement, I ordered a jade egg which arrived in a Jiffy bag. I kept finding reasons not to open it. First there was the sense that it was wrong and disgusting in some deep moral way. Then there was the fear that it would give me an infection and I'd end up in A&E feeling mortified as I explained I had stuck a stone up my vagina. I shoved it under my bed and ignored it.

I felt sad and ashamed – of what I didn't know.

Pussy puts forward the idea that in order to reach true womanhood and step into our full selves, we have to prioritize pleasure.

In theory I was all for it.

In reality I couldn't do it.

3

Sisterhood

Pussy had unsettled me in ways I did not expect. It had shone a light on dark, gnarly feelings I didn't know I had about being a woman, about my body, about my sexuality . . . about, well, my bits.

The idea of celebrating myself as a woman and allowing pleasure felt wrong in some deep way. It felt like going against everything I'd been taught but hadn't realized I'd been taught.

'Doing this work brings up a lot of stuff,' Daisy had said. 'There's a lot of shame and trauma around our vaginas.'

'I don't have trauma – nothing bad has happened to me.'

'But collectively, in society, there's trauma.'

I didn't know what she meant and I didn't want to think about anything to do with trauma or my pussy. Enough. I would get back to work instead.

I was writing an article about sexless marriages – not my own, obviously – and the printer wouldn't work. I switched it off and on again, took out the wires and put them back in. It kept telling me the printer was not connected, but it was connected.

I swore at the grey box under my desk, then felt bad. Nobody died, I told myself. Calm down.

I did this anytime I got angry: I told myself I had no reason to be angry. That it wasn't nice to be angry. I suppressed my emotions. If anyone asked me how I was it was always 'fine'.

Fine, fine, fine.

Thomashauer says that most women are like a grand piano who only ever play one note: middle C. In order to feel fully alive, we need to get used to playing the whole piano – high and low notes. We need to feel all our feelings. Our rage, our sadness, our jealousy, our excitement, our fears, our grief . . . let them all hang out.

We can do this with something called 'swamping'.

Swamping is when you put on loud angry music and just go for it. You fling yourself around the room, you rant and rave and cry and punch a pillow and let it all out. Reg docs this naked – of course she does – and sometimes with a bin bag on. If you feel rubbish, she says, why not look like it too?

Fuck it, why not?

I stopped working and googled 'best angry songs' instead. I found a website listing '11 Rage Anthems to Listen to When You're Angry'. I opened the door under the sink and pulled out a bin bag, tore a hole in it, put it over my head and stomped around the flat to Rage Against the Machine.

I caught sight of myself in my bedroom mirror – woolly hat, ski socks and bin bag – I looked ridiculous, but so what? Fuck it. I stomped my feet and punched the air and gnashed my teeth and gurned with anger. And God, I was angry . . . but not just at the printer.

I was angry with the world. Angry at myself for being so uptight. Angry at all the time I'd wasted hating my body. Angry that the first time I looked at myself, I had white hair.

Angry that I'd believed that this part of my body was bad and wrong. Angry at how hard I found it to allow myself pleasure. Angry that I was still a repressed Catholic school-girl at heart. I was angry with the nuns. Angry with my mum for not showing me another way. But then I felt guilty at this anger. I loved my mum. She'd done her best. I'd had a great life. I had no right to be angry. Anger felt ungrateful and wrong.

Kelis's song 'I Hate You So Much Right Now' came on and I mouthed the words, but I was directing them at myself. I hated myself for being so uptight, for feeling like a scared twelve-year-old instead of a forty-year-old woman. I hated myself for being such a prude. For not being a sexual woman of the world like Daisy. I wanted to shout the words, but I worried about the neighbours. Then I got angry at that. At how much of my life was spent in fear of doing anything wrong or bothering anyone. Don't make a noise! Stay quiet! Don't disturb anyone!

I felt hot tears in my eyes.

I repeated the words *I hate you so much right now* in a whisper. But I hated the hate in me. Hate was ugly. Nice girls didn't hate. Instead they pushed their feelings down until it made them sick and sad.

More music came on – Linkin Park, Eminem, angry men who felt they were perfectly entitled to rage, and to build whole careers out of it. What happens when women do that? Huh? We're accused of being mad, or on our periods.

I wanted more angry women. I went to Spotify and put on Martha Wainright's 'Bloody Mother Fucking Asshole'.

All these years of pleasing, endless pleasing. I was so tired of it.

The anger kept coming. Energy pulsed through my body, and I realized how much energy it had taken to repress my feelings. Fuck that.

As I stomped on the floor, the door opened and Daisy

walked in. With anyone else I would have stopped and felt embarrassed, but with her I kept going. Without a word she dropped her bags and started stomping too.

We screamed the title over and over again, together.

Regena Tomashauer is big on sisterhood. Not the sibling kind – the we're-all-in-it-together-as-women kind. 'Together is the only way for any of us to hit our maximum potential,' she writes. In New York she held big events for hundreds of women with pink T-shirts and feather boas.

None of this appealed.

I was one of three daughters who went to an all-girls school from the age of four to seventeen. My whole life was like a hen do without the glow-in-the-dark penis straws – or strippers for that matter. I had an allergic reaction to sisterhood talk, along with terms like 'girl boss' and 'you do you, hun' endearments.

A few months earlier, I'd been invited to listen to a talk at a women-only workspace and I'd turned it down. The whole idea of being in a women-only space (where – I assumed – rich white women spent hundreds of pounds a month to sit on armchairs and type on laptops surrounded by millennial-pink tiles and palm trees) . . . well, it repelled.

'I don't want to be with a load of women in a room complimenting each other on their outfits,' I'd said to the friend who asked me. She looked taken aback. 'That's sexist,' she'd said.

She was right. I felt ashamed.

Which is why I had signed up to a women's circle. Again, it was Daisy who had alerted me to the fact that there were dozens of women's circles all around London. Also known as goddess circles, new moon circles or red tent gatherings, these monthly meet-ups were a place for women to come together to talk, dance or rest.

I read articles claiming that these get-togethers were now the new yoga, with the likes of Jennifer Aniston holding monthly goddess gatherings at her home. Apparently Jen and her friends sat cross-legged on the living-room floor, passing around a beechwood talking stick decorated with feathers and charms. *A talking stick?*

It sounded like new-age Goop-ery but the articles told me that women have been sitting together cross-legged in circles since the dawn of time. In biblical times women would gather in a tent during their periods to rest and bleed and share lessons about sex and childbirth (hence 'red tent').

In the Sixties, consciousness-raising circles gave women the chance to share their personal experiences, and in so doing, they learned that what they thought were personal problems were in fact experiences shared by many, and often the result of sexism. These women felt emboldened to make a stand, both in their personal lives and in feminist marches, to fight for equal pay and the right to legal abortion. Women's circles had, in many ways, changed the world.

And we still had a long way to go.

I sat cross-legged on a faux sheepskin rug. Plinky plonky music, the smell of sage burning. Of course. Everyone else's eyes were closed, so I closed mine too.

'When we connect with our divine feminine,' a woman with a soft voice was saying, 'we connect with our deeper knowing.'

We were sitting in a circle in a hip room in East London. Rose petals were arranged in the centre of the room, surrounding a single rose in a vase and a burning candle.

We were being told to breathe in, 'all the way down to your womb space'. I felt itchy and scratchy and I wanted to get out. The idea of a womb space felt dark and gnarly, and . . . anyway, where *was* my womb? How did I breathe into it? I started to feel panicked. This reminded me of being in my first year at school and being asked to draw a yo-yo, but I didn't know what a yo-yo was. I tried to look at my neighbour's drawing and copy it, but felt the hot shame of now knowing what a yo-yo was as I drew a wonky circle with a line coming out of the top of it. Forty years later, I remember her name: Sophia Smith.

Why didn't I know where my womb was? But I didn't know where my liver was, either. Or my kidneys . . . how was I so ignorant of my body?

'You might want to put your hands to your womb as you breathe in,' the teacher said. Her voice was soft and slow and whispery – it was driving me mad. Speak up, woman!

I opened my eyes to see what the other women were doing. They had their hands at the bottom of their tummies, making a diamond shape. All of them had their eyes closed.

They were all younger and hotter than me. I bet they all did yoga. And had crystals and no cellulite.

I copied them.

Someone let out a long sigh. Attention-seeker.

'Would anyone like to share what came up for them?' the teacher asked after finishing the meditation. 'For those of you who have not been with us before, a reminder that there is no pressure to share anything. This is a safe space to say whatever comes up for you, and your silence is welcome. Your presence is a gift.'

Me and my womb – wherever it was – sat in silence.

———

When the 'sharing' started, we were 'invited' to listen to each other in silence, without offering advice or giving reassurance. We were just to hold each 'sister' in 'loving presence'.

The first woman spoke in a way that suggested she'd done these things before. She had all the jargon. She wanted 'to drop down and meet herself', and to 'work through' some long-term health issues that she believed stemmed from 'unexpressed grief'. She irritated me. Who talked like that? And why did she have to come to a room full of other women to meet herself? Surely she could have just looked in the mirror.

The woman next to her spoke with her head down, saying that she worked in a male-dominated industry and felt like she needed to spend more time with women. Boring.

Then a young woman in black was ripping tissues into shreds as she talked about caring for her eighty-year-old father. She had an older boyfriend and he repulsed her. She wondered if she hated both him and her father. She also wondered if she was sexually attracted to women. Ooh, now that was more interesting.

Another talked about the death of her sister when she was six. Thirty years later she kept dreaming about her sister.

A very beautiful woman who looked about thirty started to speak. At first I didn't hear what she was saying, I was too busy envying her tanned skin and silky hair. I'd seen her take off Acne boots on the way in, and she had a Chanel handbag. She must have been rich as well as beautiful – your basic nightmare, to quote *When Harry Met Sally*. I imagined what life must be like if you were that good-looking.

'I fuck men I don't want to fuck,' she said. 'And then I feel like shit. And then I watch porn. Violent porn. I want to be hurt, and sometimes I put myself in situations where that happens.'

Oh.

Eventually the woman next to me stopped talking and tapped my knee to signal it was my turn.

'Um, I don't know what to say, really . . .' As I looked at their faces looking at me, I felt hot with self-consciousness. I imagined them judging me. I imagined them thinking I was a loser, a fat loser with no boyfriend . . . hang on. Why was I thinking that?

Instantly, I knew why this circle made me so uncomfortable. It reminded me of being a teenager at sleepovers. All night the talk was of boys, who had done what with whom. The 'never have I ever' game would be played and I would fall silent. Only I had never done anything with anyone.

Every time I was with a group of women I was thirteen again. Thirteen and the sad weirdo who hadn't kissed anyone.

'I'm sorry, I feel quite tense when I'm in a room of women like this,' I said. They kept looking, with passive, open faces.

I waited for someone to laugh. They didn't.

I didn't know what else to say so I patted the woman next to me, as a signal that I had finished talking.

The next woman spoke. 'I just left my husband of twenty-two years . . . A friend sent me a link to a YouTube video about coercive control and it was the first time I understood what he'd been doing to me.'

She paused.

'All those years I knew something was wrong and I didn't have the language to describe what it was – then I watched that video and it was all there.'

We listened in silence.

'As soon as I saw it, I couldn't stay. I made a plan and got the kids out. We found a safe place to stay. I couldn't have them thinking that was normal . . . how he was.'

You could hear a pin drop.

'Once I left I found out he'd put recording devices in our house, he was recording all our conversations . . . I felt so stupid, that I hadn't seen it before—'

We were all meant to sit in silence and just listen to each other, but one woman couldn't help herself. 'You're not stupid! This is what they do – abusers, they make you think it's your fault. Or that you're making it up. It's not your problem. It's theirs. That takes guts what you did, getting out.' She spoke with the urgency of experience.

'Thank you,' the first woman replied. 'Once I knew, I couldn't stay. My soul would have died.'

The weight of that sentence hit me. *My soul would have died.* I wondered how many women were living with souls that had died.

'Did any of your friends see what he was doing?' asked another woman. 'Try to warn you?'

'He made sure I didn't have much contact with people. I'd lost a lot of friends by the end.'

'This is why women need places like this . . . Places where it's just women,' somebody else said.

The teacher asked us to take each other's hands and close our eyes. The woman on my right had a soft, gentle hold; her skin felt cool and moisturized. On my left, the anxious grip of bony fingers that were shaking slightly. I held her tight.

After a herbal tea break we were invited to find space to move around in. I went to the furthest corner and closed my eyes. At first a slow, wafty track played and we were told to 'be with whatever is there'. I closed my eyes and swayed and it felt nice.

'You might want to put your hand to your heart to welcome yourself here, in this body, in a room with your sisters . . .'

I put my hand to my heart and felt my eyes dampen.

'Send some love to this beautiful body and soul who is always there for you, always available, even when we ignore it or punish it.'

A fat tear ran down my cheek.

'And now I invite you to explore your depths, your darkness, your shadow . . . Really meet yourself in the feelings that we so often suppress – our anger, our rage, our fear, our jealousy . . .'

The music started to intensify, with a pounding beat. I stomped my feet as I had done in my kitchen, stomping out the anger, the ugliness, the stuckness I often felt. This time I wasn't worried about other people. I let out a shout and it felt so good I did it again. Other women followed me.

The music changed to a more sad, sweepy song with a tinkling piano. I kept my eyes closed and swayed slowly and found tears streaming down my face.

'Welcome your grief,' the teacher was saying. 'Welcome it – your grief is sacred. It is not just your grief, it is the grief of your mother and your mother's mother, and her ancestors . . . we hold it all in us, and we must honour our grief for a world that has devalued the feminine.'

I thought about the beautiful woman wanting people to hurt her, and the woman whose partner had hurt her in ways I could not understand. Why did people do that to each other? Why did men do that? Why? I cried for all the women of the world who had been abused. So many. I thought of the woman who had lost her sister, the woman struggling to make her way in a male-dominated office, the woman caring for her older father . . .

I thought about my mum being taught not to love herself. I thought of myself being taught not to love myself. All this stuff that I didn't know I'd been carrying now felt unbearably heavy.

I found myself on the floor crouched down and crying with exhaustion, and I felt an arm on my back. The Acne-boots woman was crouched down next to me, rubbing my back gently.

Then the music seemed to lighten and almost tinkle, a piano was doing something that made it seem like sunshine on a rainy day, and my head and neck straightened up so that I looked up to the high ceiling of this old church, and I felt hope again.

For the first time I looked around the room at the women who were each dancing in their own way, some with eyes closed, some eyes open. Some moving and spinning, some still . . . I wasn't judging them now, or comparing. I was smiling at their beauty.

God, women were beautiful.

Eventually the music changed again and I recognized the song that came on . . . it was Beyonce's 'Run The World (Girls)'. I smiled at the cheesiness of it but soon the smile turned into a grin and I was shouting the words out loud and my eyes were open and I was dancing and flinging my arms in the air and shaking my hips with all the women around me and it was glorious.

One woman had taken her top off and was jumping up and down in a black lace bra with her eyes squeezed shut as she shouted the words. She had a scar running up her tummy and one of her breasts had been removed. She looked magnificent.

The music stopped and we were invited to close our eyes, and I smiled to be in this room with other women.

'Take this moment to be with yourself,' the teacher was saying. 'To be with yourself and feel yourself as a woman.'

My heart was pounding. My face was grinning. I felt alive. Inspired. Uplifted.

'You might want to put your hands to your womb again and see if it has a message for you.'

I put my hands in the diamond shape on my tummy, as I'd seen the other women do. *Do you have a message for me, womb?* I asked.

I am here, it said.

I beamed on the bus home. Although I'd hated it at first, by the end, being in a room full of women talking and dancing felt . . . right.

I tried to understand why it had been so different to my evenings with friends. Perhaps it was different because we were not allowed to offer advice, to fix or reassure. Our job was just to listen no matter what was being said. That felt good, to speak and be heard, with no solutions offered. I liked that at no point did any of us revert to the usual 'my bum is too big' spiel or make jokes. This was more real than that.

I thought of the woman who put her hand on me and teared up again at the beauty of that small gesture of care and, well, sisterhood.

It was something I hadn't known I needed, but I did: the care and acceptance of other women. But I already had that in my life, surely?

I had spent my life in female-only environments, so why was this the first time I was experiencing this feeling? I could see how often my guard was up, how often I didn't say the thing that was really bothering me, for fear I'd be taking up time or that I'd seem silly. Even though I was surrounded by wonderful women, there was always a bit of me that feared their judgement.

Thomashauer explains that we are taught not to trust other women, taught that 'woman are backbiting, envious, catty, emotionally unstable, hysterical, premenstrual and unreasonable. We have been taught that, given the chance, women will take each other down.'

I didn't know if I believed all that – though maybe on some level I did? At the very least, I had the same antipathy for other women that I held for myself as a woman. I also, if I was being honest, saw them as competition. But for what – jobs? Men? Both?

I thought about how quickly I had compared myself to the other women in the room, instantly clocking who was prettier, thinner, better dressed than me. I noticed how quick I had been to criticize women I considered more beautiful, more clever. Being a woman meant always being judged or feeling judged. Not just by men, but by each other as well.

But it doesn't have to be that way.

I vowed to be a better cheerleader to the women in my life. I vowed to myself that I would never say another bad word about another woman.

On the way out I'd seen that one of the women had a tote bag with the slogan *Feminism encourages women to leave their husbands, practice witchcraft, destroy capitalism and become lesbians.*

That could be the next stage.

It was Rachel's birthday and she was having Sunday lunch in a pub. I arrived early and found her sister at the table. She was wearing a bright purple blouse, huge hoops and was reading a book. I gave her a hug and told her how gorgeous she looked.

'Oh God, don't, I'm a state. I put bronzer on on the bus – do I look like a dry-roasted peanut?'

I told her she didn't but that it was a good line.

Rachel arrived with her old school friend Amy, with apologies about being late. I knew that Amy had just been promoted and I congratulated her. 'Yeah, let's see how long it lasts.'

And so began a lunch in which each of us, in the name of good manners and banter, took turns to put ourselves down.

Wrinkles. Weight. Excessive drinking. Shit mothering. My mad hair and embarrassing quest to find sexual liberation by looking at my pussy in a mirror.

Thomashauer explains that women bond over woes rather than strengths because we see each other as competition, and so we parade our problems as a way of saying *look, I'm not a threat to you.* We talk about our terrible day at work, make jokes about our chin hairs and generally put ourselves down instead of telling everyone about our promotion or the great sex we just had. We do this to be likeable, but this communication has a damaging effect – it bonds women to their pain rather than their potential.

I related.

I'd spent my life putting myself down – made a career out of it, even. I wanted to get the criticisms in before anyone else did, and had been brought up with the idea that nobody likes a show off and that humility was charming. But was it?

I'd started to feel there was nothing endearing about my need to put myself down like I had self-deprecation Tourette's. Not only did it put other people under pressure to say, 'Don't be silly, you're fabulous', I could see that it was hurting me. If you call yourself a mess often enough do you start to believe it? But not only was it affecting me, it was also playing into the culture that says that if a woman is visible or successful she'd better make jokes about her crazy hair or crap love life. This was hurting all of us. And keeping us down.

Instead of comparing woes, Thomashauer suggests an approach called The Holy Trinity.

1. Brag about something you've done well.
2. Share something you're grateful for.
3. Describe something you desire.

I asked the table if they'd be up for trying it. At first we found it hard to find things to brag about. It felt unnatural and clunky.

'I brag that I pay my rent by myself in one of the most expensive cities in the world,' I said.

'You can do better than that,' Rachel said.

'OK, I brag that my writing is read all around the world, and makes people feel better.' They all clapped, and I felt my cheeks fire up.

Amy said she was proud of being the only female director in her firm. We clapped again.

Her sister bragged that even though she was knackered she'd done a run that morning.

The whole energy of the table changed. Thomashauer says that bragging in itself is a kind of activism. She believes that the early feminist movement was based on anger, but that now is the time for a feminism fuelled by happiness and celebration of being a woman.

We took it in turn to do our gratitudes, and they came more easily. We were all grateful for the people in our lives and for good health.

Finally, time to name our desires.

I hated the word 'desire'. It sounded like a word used to sell perfume. 'Desire', a sultry voice would say over a shot of a naked couple on a beach, 'the new parfum by Calvin Klein. Want More. Want It All . . .'

Admitting a desire felt exposing. Thoughts like *Who do you think you are?* came into my head. What was the point in wanting things that would never happen? I felt greedy for wanting . . . but at the same time, naming desires felt thrilling.

My answer came quickly: 'I desire lots of great sex and a nice house!' I laughed as I said it. But I actually *did* desire both of those things. Why did I need to laugh about it?

Rachel's sister desired more time to herself, and to let go of the feeling that she always needed to be doing something productive.

Rachel said simply: 'I want a child. I've decided I'm going to freeze my eggs.'

4

But What About Children?

There was quiet around the table as Rachel spoke.

'The stats are shitty and it costs a fortune, but I don't see what other choice I have. I'm done with going on dates looking for a father for my children . . .' she said. 'I've found a clinic and I'm going to do it.'

'That's great,' I said straight away. The others didn't. 'So how does it work?' I asked, filling the silence.

'You take hormones that make you make lots of eggs, then they take them out and freeze them so that you can use them later,' Rachel said.

'So you'd use them if you met someone and you'd have younger eggs?' Amy asked.

'Yeah, and if I don't meet anyone I could get a donor's sperm and have a baby on my own.'

'Do you really want to do it on your own?' Amy asked.

'It's not a matter of wanting it,' Rachel snapped. 'It's just the situation I'm in.'

'You're brave,' I chimed in, wanting to be supportive.

'I'm not,' she replied. 'I just want children.'

'You know it's a lot to do on your own . . .' Amy said.

'Yes, of course I know that,' Rachel said. Her cheeks were getting pink.

'I support you and whatever you want to do, but I'm

just saying it's a lot – even with two of you it's a lot,' said Amy.

'I know that,' Rachel repeated.

'How much does it cost?' I wanted to change direction.

'Four thousand a pop. I'm going to do three rounds because apparently some eggs when they're defrosted won't be good enough to fertilise – so that's twelve thousand pounds.'

'Well, fuck it, that's what savings are for,' I said. 'And at least this gives you options.'

On the train home I thought about Rachel spending so much money on having a child, or even the potential of having a child. As she said, there were no guarantees. I didn't have that kind of cash, but even if I did, I didn't know if I'd spend it on getting my eggs frozen.

I could think of so many other things I'd rather do with it: book a plane to California, buy a trouser suit, give mum a chunk of money, pay off Daisy's credit cards. Pay off my own credit cards.

I thought about Amy's warnings. Would it be too much for Rachel to do on her own? Amy had separated from her partner but they shared custody and expenses. Her ex's parents were hands-on. There was a support network.

Rachel had her sister, but her parents lived abroad and I lived on the other side of London. But if anyone could do it, she could.

Could I? Would I?

In my mid-thirties an older, childless friend had told me that when I was forty a bomb would go off and I would be obsessed with the desire to have a child.

So far, no bomb.

I wondered if I was a late developer, or in denial. I

wondered if my ambivalence came from not having met the love of my life. Maybe if I fell madly in love, I'd want their children? Or maybe I avoided falling madly in love because I didn't want anyone's children.

When I visited friends with children, I never came home wishing I had what they had. When people talked about physically yearning to have a child and 'ovaries exploding', I couldn't relate.

'Do you want children?' I asked Daisy that night.

'Yes,' she said. It surprised me. 'I'd love to have the family I never had, but I don't think it's realistic. I'd have to meet the right person . . . which probably isn't going to happen and anyway, even if it did, I don't know if I'd be a good mum. I can barely look after myself. I was on a train the other day and a baby was screaming and I thought, no way – I'll get a cat instead.'

I laughed, but I felt sad for her. Her childhood had been a difficult one, with a dad who wasn't around and a mother who may as well not have been. 'Anyway,' she said. 'I don't think it's right with the world the way it is – you'd be bringing them into an environmental apocalypse.'

'Oh, yeah.' I hadn't thought about that side of things.

'What about you?' she asked me.

'I don't think I want them.'

'Why not?'

'I don't know if there's a reason why – I just don't. I don't have any desire to have a mini-me in the world.'

'Don't say that.'

'I'm not saying I think it would be a bad thing – I just honestly don't have that urge.' But even as I said this, I doubted myself . . .

I had bought Sheila Heti's *Motherhood* a few months earlier because of a quote I'd read on the back of the book:

'Whether I want kids is a secret I keep from myself – it is the greatest secret I keep from myself.'

Exactly.

After the Rachel news, I picked up the book and read it in one sitting, underlining vigorously. The circular narrative infuriated some reviewers but I related to the feeling of going around and around the topic, thinking you were making a decision on something while really you were waiting for the option to be taken off the table.

This was one of the passages I underlined:

'She doesn't want a baby – but her body doesn't believe her. On some level, no one believes her. On some level, she doesn't even believe herself.' Exactly. I didn't believe myself when I said I didn't think I wanted children. I didn't believe other women either. You'll change your mind, I thought.

Then there was this:

'There is sadness in not wanting the things that give so many other people their life's meaning.' Yes – that was it!

It felt lonely not doing what my friends were doing. Until recently we were on the same path. Even when they got married and bought houses and stuff, we still hung out. But when the babies came, things changed.

Maybe that was the issue. Not whether I wanted children or marriage, but the fact that I no longer fitted in with the people around me. With every passing year I felt more at odds with life's norms, and a part of me thought I should desperately row back and try to get it right. Get back on the path everyone else was on.

———

'Do you think I'll regret not having children?'

'There are many ways to live your life,' my therapist said.

I looked out of the window at the walled garden behind her. I wondered how much her house had cost. I found myself having the usual thoughts about how my therapist had done it 'right'. She had got married, had children, saved money, bought a house with a garden . . . I had a rented flat, no partner, no children and an ever-dwindling bank balance.

She kept looking at me, rubbing her slippered feet together. I wondered how old she was.

'You have children, don't you?' I asked her.

'Yes.'

'And are they the best thing that ever happened to you?'

'Quite often they are a disappointment,' she said.

I was shocked.

'Oh,' I said.

'It's important that women are honest about motherhood. Very often they are not.'

I thought of the woman at mum's book club.

When my book came out, they'd invited me to come and speak. I'd expected the stiff-upper-lip generation to ride roughshod over my dreams to make an already good life better, but they were sympathetic. They talked about children and grandchildren with mental health issues and the worry they felt about the state of the world. They asked me about the Greek and whether I'd got out of debt. They asked me if I wanted to get married and have children. I'd said I didn't know.

'There's no rush for all that,' one of them had said.

'No need to do it at all!' another added, a tall woman in a yellow Pringle jumper with cropped white hair. 'I should never have been a mother.'

She had been an academic at a time when women were not

academics – and her devotion to work meant her kids were neglected. 'Neither of them talk to me now,' she said.

'Do you know why I had children?' mum had asked. I perked up. For a second I imagined that maybe she would talk about how she couldn't wait to hold her own baby, or how she'd always known that she was meant to be a mother. But no. The reason mum had us?

'Because I got pregnant!' she said.

The group laughed because it was the truth. In her generation children were not these carefully planned beings, who came into your life only when you'd built a career and taken nice trips – children were just something that happened. Something you accepted and did your best with, but not something you necessarily chose or even wanted.

I had a choice. Just as I had a choice about whether to get married or not. All these choices were wonderful, and exhausting.

'Not everyone is built to parent, and the aunty role is very important. It sounds like you're involved with your friends' children's lives,' my therapist said.

I nodded. I was, but not as much as I felt I should be. I felt guilty about that. A free-floating guilt – as a free, single woman, should I have been using my spare time to help my friends with their kids? But I didn't actually want to spend my non-working hours as an unpaid babysitter. Was that selfish? It was, wasn't it?

'And there are different ways to contribute to the world – you could say you do that through your work,' my therapist said.

'Yeah, but I worry that my writing is just ego, or a way of compensating for other things that are missing. Anyway, this whole conversation – about babies – might be pointless.

I'm single and I doubt I even could have kids at this point.' I said.

'It might be worth finding out,' she said.

That night I googled fertility testing and a few sites came up. One told me the reasons I should test my hormones and fertility today, alerting me to the fact that 88 per cent of my eggs may be gone by the time I hit thirty.

Great, thanks for that.

At forty, what would I have left? One and a half hard-boiled eggs?

There are many causes of female infertility, they told me, and this kit would help me find out if any of them applied to me. (What about male fertility? Why was it always women's fault?) Next fun fact: 64 per cent of us have at least one hormone out of range; one in ten has polycystic ovarian syndrome . . . God, this was depressing. I was so bored of being given stats about our fertility dropping off a cliff and career women leaving it too late.

But what was 'too late'? Catherine Gray reckons that those figures about fertility falling off a cliff at thirty-five were from a study from 1700s France. She said in the UK two thousand babies a year are born to mothers over forty-five. So maybe there *was* time?

I remembered something in Sheila Heti's *Motherhood*: 'I thought about how unfair it was that she and I had to think about having kids – that we had to sit here talking about it, feeling like if we didn't have children, we would always regret it. It suddenly seemed like a huge conspiracy to keep women in their thirties – when you finally have some brains and some skills and experience – from doing anything useful with them at all. It is hard to when such a large portion of your mind, at any given time, is preoccupied with the possibility – a question that didn't seem to preoccupy the drunken men at all.'

I wondered how much time and energy my friends and I had spent going around in circles on these things – marriage, relationships, children. Too much. Way, way too much.

And so I went back to ignoring the baby question.

5

Tantra

For years I've had a stress dream that involves me in a department store going up and down escalators tugging on the white shirt I'm wearing in the hope that I can cover my knickers, because in this dream I accidentally left the house without anything on my bottom half.

Now I was experiencing a new variation of this dream – the variation being that it wasn't a dream.

I had, against every fibre of my being, decided to accept an invitation to a tantra retreat, to write about it for a magazine. I'd never been invited to something like this before, and the fact that the email had landed as I was exploring love and, in theory at least, sex, did probably count as a sign. Daisy was certain it did.

I googled the teacher and read articles about how her workshops helped people set boundaries and give themselves permission to enjoy pleasure. 'Setting boundaries' sounded safe – and fully dressed – so I was clinging to it . . . and *Pussy* had shown me I needed help on the pleasure front.

Daisy was all for it, Gemma too. Sarah and Rachel were not. I sent Rachel a link to an article which featured a photograph of a group of people sitting cross-legged in a circle while a woman with red hair stood in the middle talking to them.

'Look at what they're wearing . . .' she texted. She was put off by their fashion choices while I was just relieved to see they were wearing clothes. 'Don't do it,' said Sarah, 'it'll be full of creeps.'

And at first I thought she was right. A man wearing patch-work pants opened the door when I arrived at Florence House.

'Welcome,' he said, and I was both transfixed and disgusted by a tiny tuft of hair under his bottom lip, shaped like a tri-angle. Gross.

'I'm . . .' he paused for a second, 'I'm – er, Jay,' he said, like he was trying the name on for size. I kept looking at his tuft. How vain and insecure do you have to be to shape your facial hair into that? And he was also wearing a necklace – a shiny black stone on a black string of leather. Pretentious hippy bullshit.

'Would you like a hug?' he asked.

'No,' I said. Inwardly. Outwardly, I grinned and said, 'Sure.'

He opened his arms and made a 'mmm' sound as he gripped me, and instead of going in and straight out, he re-arranged himself so that his hips were in contact with mine, and his tummy and chest. I stepped to move away but he stayed there, holding me, 'mmm'ing, his tummy inflating and deflating against me.

When he released me, eighty-five years later, he let out a sigh.

'Ah, that felt good . . .' he said, drilling holes in my eyes. It was like he was playing a game of chicken.

His skin was good. Obnoxiously good.

'Do you work here?' I asked.

'No, I'm a participant, taking another step on my journey . . .'

I thought of mum's loathing of the word 'journey'. No, don't think of mum.

Tufty-hair guy – 'er, Jay' – pointed me towards a stern-looking man sitting behind a pine table with a clipboard. He checked my address, asked in a German accent whether I had any food allergies and gave me my room number, with smile-free efficiency. I told him I didn't eat mushrooms but I wasn't allergic. 'I just don't like them,' I said.

He did not seem fascinated by this insight into my world.

'Please, also, sign this,' he said, handing me a piece of paper saying, amongst other things, that should any sexual activity take place it would be a good idea to use a condom.

Condoms?

Condoms!

We weren't actually going to be having sex, were we?

No. We couldn't be.

I made my way to my room, where an older woman with hair the colour of honey was unpacking. She was wearing turquoise leggings and a low-cut top. After introducing myself to her, I asked, 'Did you see that condom bit in the disclaimer?'

'I will not be putting any condoms on anyone!' she said.

'Good, me neither.' I felt relieved.

'Did you bring your blindfold?' she asked.

'What?'

'It said we should bring sarongs and blindfolds.'

'I didn't see that – why do we need a blindfold?' I said, panicked.

'No idea.'

I felt sick. Physically sick.

'I only came because a friend recommended it, but she wouldn't tell me anything about it,' my roommate said.

'But did she say it was good?'

'It must have been. She signed up for the eighteen-month training.'

'And is she . . . can you see a difference in her?'

'The other week we were supposed to go the cinema and she called to cancel and she didn't even make an excuse or pretend she was sick, she just said, "I don't feel like the cinema today." '

'Wow.'

We paused to take in this radical behaviour.

'I was livid, actually,' she said. 'We can't all just do what we want, can we?'

'I don't know,' I said.

We went down for a dinner of vegetable dhal on country kitchen pine tables. I was too scared to eat. Instead I looked around to see if everyone was a pervert. They didn't seem to be – though there were two more men wearing necklaces.

After dinner we met in a large, carpeted room, with French windows along one side, facing into darkness.

Some kind of dance music was playing. I moved from side to side with a rictus grin on my face. My roommate moved from side to side next to me. We smiled at each other. Yup, just keep smiling, be cool.

A man with a tie-dye T-shirt with an elephant on it had his eyes closed and his arms raised to the sky. A slim woman with dark hair twirled around him like a spinning top.

The music stopped and a woman with a Madonna headset microphone started talking. She was pale-skinned, red-haired and dressed head-to-toe in blue. She stood with her feet apart, her knees slightly bent. I assumed she was Jan Day, our teacher, but I didn't hear her introduce herself. Instead she got

straight to it, inviting the men to go to one end of the room
and the women to the other.

'Now close your eyes,' she said, 'and take a deep breath
and think: How do you feel in this body as a woman? How
do you feel as a man?'

I closed my eyes and breathed.

How does it feel to be in this body as a woman? My thoughts,
as usual, did a mental inventory of everything I hated about
my body. My fat, saggy, dimpled bum. Then they went to my
tummy which, despite not having had dinner, still felt heavy
after eating a Pret club and crisps on the train.

Then I felt angry at myself. *Get over it!*

'Now you are invited to open your eyes and to move, as
slowly as you'd like, towards the other side of the room,' said
the teacher. 'See how it feels to be a woman faced with a man,
and a man faced with a woman.'

I felt the stress rising. I didn't want to be a woman faced
with a man, I wanted to be a woman safe on the side of the
room with the other women. Why hadn't I just signed up for
more women's circles? I hung by the back wall, but the other
women were moving forward and I didn't want to hang back
on my own. I stepped forward.

A man with huge brown eyes walked towards me and
I willed myself not to run away. My heart pounded and
my throat felt tight. His eyes worked through me like lasers.
What was he staring at? And why was it so stressful just to
look at him?

If I looked away I knew he would see how scared I was,
and I didn't want him to see that. But his looking was freak-
ing me out. What did it mean? Did it mean he fancied me?
Did I want him to fancy me? Or not? Did I have to do something now?

He was wearing white linen trousers with the cleanest

white T-shirt I'd ever seen. He looked like a tantric physiother-apist. I could never go out with a man dressed like that. For a second, I felt relieved. There you go, I didn't fancy him – now he had no power over me! Then just to prove it, I walked away from him before he could walk away from me. Tri-umph! I had rejected him before he had rejected me.

'Notice your patterns,' the teacher was saying. 'Notice when you stay and you really want to go, or when you go and you would really like to have stayed. Notice if you cut short the connection out of fear.'

Another set of eyes were in front me now, belonging to a white-haired man wearing a colourful shirt with pine-apples on it. He smiled and I smiled back. His eyes twinkled and my heart slowed down. He was grinning now and I was grinning back. I could feel a drop of sweat roll down the side of my face. I wished I didn't sweat so much. He was sweating too. I felt safe with this man, but I didn't want him to get any ideas. I didn't want him to think that I fan-cied him.

I nodded in what I hoped was an acknowledgment of our time together and stepped away, bumping, literally, into a tall man with green eyes, probably early thirties. He was wearing a white T-shirt and tracksuit bottoms. I panicked.

He was good-looking. My cheeks burned, and before I could go through the full list of reasons I would not be good enough for a man like this – too fat! Too ginger! Gaps in my teeth! Big scar on my leg! Shit in bed! – he nodded, as if he'd read my mind and was in full agreement. He walked away. I felt a tickle at the back of my throat and my eyes sting with tears. I'd been rejected by a total stranger. A man whose name I did not know. And it cut me to the core.

———

That night I lay awake in bed, certain that I had made a huge mistake by coming.

The next morning, after a night of fitful sleep, we returned to the carpeted room, which was now filled with mattresses. Hippy music was playing. The German man from the check-in was telling everyone to find a mattress and put our sarongs over the mattress. We could buy a blindfold if we didn't have one.

I picked a mattress in the back of the room and laid out the red sarong with a giant parrot that Daisy had lent me. I looked out of the French doors onto the garden. In daylight I could see the golf course next door. I wondered if maybe I'd even prefer golf to being here.

The music came on loud and we were told to put our blindfolds on and shake our bodies. Shake, shake, shake. Like a rag doll. 'Shake up from the ground!' the German man was telling us. Whatever that meant. I shook my legs, backside, arms. People around me were making odd noises. I kept shaking.

Then the music changed into something more drum-like, and we were told to get down on the floor to express our 'animal nature' – oh god. What?

I didn't have an animal nature. I went to convent school.

The room filled with grunting and groaning, whimpering and wailing, shouting and swearing . . . I sneaked a look under my blindfold to see what people were doing. I wished I hadn't. They were hurling pillows against the mattresses, ripping off their clothes and humping their pillows.

I couldn't hump my pillow. I just couldn't. It's not how I was raised.

I imagined the teacher looking at me, taking notes on the sexually repressed one in the corner. When the music changed to plinky plonky fairy dust, I was relieved. It was time for the lying down breathing bit. That I could do.

After a breakfast that I couldn't eat, we were back in the room, sitting in a circle. We were invited to have a couple of minutes each to say why we were there. People talked about different things: divorce, sexless marriages, finding it hard to connect with others, body image issues . . . some just wanted to explore their sexuality more.

I was unnerved by how frequently and freely people were using the word 'sexuality'. I imagined that they were sexually liberated people of the world. I was sure I would be the least sexually experienced person here.

One of the necklace-wearers – a lab technician from Ipswich – announced to the group that he was 'available for hugs'.

Our teacher spoke a bit about tantra, which is said to be the oldest Eastern tradition of spiritual philosophy and prac- tice, starting more than 5,000 years ago in India. While many religions separate sexuality and spirituality, tantra doesn't. A key teaching of tantra is that nothing is impure, everything is one and sacred, all existence is a manifestation of the divine, and the belief that the body and the sensual experiences of the body are part of the divine rather than a distraction.

'Our sexual energy isn't only about sex,' Jan had said. 'In fact, it's not even mostly about sex. Your sexual energy is your life energy: it's the centre from which your interest in life, your joie de vivre, arises. It's the kernel of your aliveness.'

The kernel of your aliveness. I liked that.

We were asked to make groups of four: two men and two women. We were encouraged to not make a beeline to work with our 'usual types' but to be open-minded and work with people we might not usually be drawn to. My four were composed of the three people nearest me – I preferred not to make an active choice, it turned out, but go with whatever was easiest.

Jan was telling us we would take it in turns to stand in the middle and ask the others to touch us. We could say one, two or three, depending on how many people we wanted to touch us – or we could say zero.

'The aim is to find your boundaries,' said Jan in a tone that was brisk, stern and motherly at the same time. 'To explore what feels good and what doesn't. You are in control and can express dislike, or stop at any time.'

I was in a group with the white-haired man who was wearing another colourful shirt, this time with flowers on it, a woman with white, curly hair who looked like my GCSE religion teacher, and the hot, green-eyed guy. Why was he here? Surely his love life must be a breeze, looking like that?

Jan was still talking.

'For example, you might say that you are happy for your arms and face to be touched, but you do not want your breasts or genitals to be touched,' Jan explained.

What? I didn't know these people's names! Nobody was going to be touching my genitals.

'The point of this exercise is that you must never do anything you do not want to do,' said Jan. 'For some of you the most important learning will be to say no to touch, for others it will be allowing yourself to say yes, and to enjoy it.'

The religion teacher said that she would go first. She stood in the middle and we arranged ourselves in a triangle around her. 'I'm fine with you touching me everywhere,' she said, with no shame or shyness. Amazing. I guessed she wasn't actually a religion teacher.

'One,' she said, with her eyes closed. We all looked at each other and the man in the colourful shirt – who I decided looked like a Hawaiian Santa – nodded for me to touch her. I put my hand on her shoulder and started to slowly stroke the top of her arm. I worried I was doing it wrong. She kept smiling.

'Two,' came the next request. The younger guy hesitantly stepped closer and started to rub her other arm. 'Yes, please,' she said, as we smiled at each other at a job well done.

Our instructions were to say 'yes', 'no', 'please', and 'pause' or 'stop'. 'Yes' meant 'yes, please, I like that'. 'No' was a 'no, don't touch me there'. 'Please' was 'I really, really like that, more please', and 'pause' was 'I just need a second to process what's happening here'. 'Stop' meant all hands came off.

'Three, please.' Hawaiian Santa stood in front of her and stroked her hair. 'Please,' she said when the hair-stroking started. I felt embarrassed by her obvious enjoyment.

We adjusted positions so that Santa moved to stroke the back of her head and I moved to the front of her body and stroked her cheeks. She looks blissed-out, and despite the utter weirdness of this situation I surprised myself by feeling proud to make this woman I didn't know happy.

This was fun! Weird, but fun.

Next up was the hot guy. He reminded me of a guy I'd had a crush on at the local boys' school. He played rugby and guitar and was one of those effortless sex-god, musical-genius, sporty guys that could have his pick of the girls . . . goes without saying that he never picked me.

'One,' he said, and the religion teacher went in and gently traced her fingers along the side of his face, like he was a work of art. He started to breathe heavily, and I could see him swallow. 'Pause,' he said. She paused and they stood still, like musical statues.

'Two,' he said. I looked at Santa, who nodded for me to go next. I hovered beside him and felt paralysed. My heart pounded and I was worried that my shaky, sweaty hands would feel gross to him.

I plumped for his right arm, stroking it all the way down with my sticky hands. When I got to his hand, I found myself wanting to hold it. So I did. 'No,' he said, and I jumped back like I'd had an electric shock.

I had done it wrong! All my fears were founded! I didn't know how to touch a hot man!

'Three,' he said, seemingly unaware of the dagger he'd put through my heart. I moved forward again, not because I wanted to touch him but because pride had kicked in and I wanted to show everyone that his 'no' had not hurt me. I was a mature adult who could take a 'no'. Yeah, no big deal.

I went back to stroking his arm with my sweaty hands and Santa put both hands firmly on his feet. And then he seemed to breathe more steadily.

I went last. I didn't want anyone touching me, but still I said 'One', 'two', 'three', signalling all of them to go for it.

I was terrified and pretending not to be. The main game here was saving face, but I was sure everyone could see through me. Instead of enjoying the touch, it brought up all my worst thoughts about myself. They think you're a prude! They think you're shit in bed! They think you're a ginger minger! They think you're fat! They can tell you're a repressed Catholic schoolgirl who doesn't have boyfriends!

I could have said 'no' or 'stop' or 'zero', but I didn't want people to think that I was repressed, so I stood there like a frozen animal as touches came to my arms, my shoulders, my hands and my hair.

Hot guy put his hands in my hair and it felt like fingernails on a blackboard. Jan's voice kept reminding us that 'no' is not a rejection, it's simply information. 'You should never tolerate touch you do not like,' she said.

I clenched and waited for it to be over.

Afterwards we sat in a circle and started the mortifying process of talking about how that had been for us. Hot guy said he had felt very nervous and self-conscious, and that his heart was pounding and that he'd found it hard to relax. He said that at some point he felt someone hold his hand and that that was 'not necessary'. My cheeks burned.

The religion teacher talked about how beautiful it was to be touched, that she had not been touched in months, and I winced at how open she was being. Santa said something similar, but I was only listening to them through a prism of comparing and judging myself. Why did everyone seem to speak freely when I could barely speak at all?

'Lovely,' I said. 'Yeah, really nice!'

'I sensed a bit of tension,' said Santa, with kind eyes. 'I worried that perhaps you were suffering from touch that you didn't like.'

'No, not at all! It was lovely!' I said.

We left the room and I ran to the loo, feeling sick with the humiliating realization that even as I hit middle age, I was terrified of everything. Terrified of men, especially hot ones. Terrified of being rejected, terrified of not being rejected. Terrified of not knowing what to do, or of doing it – touch, sex – wrong, terrified of being seen to not know what to do.

Jan kept saying that this energy was the life force within us, but being in the presence of this life force was giving me a pain in my chest so strong I wondered if perhaps I was having a mild heart attack.

Imagine that, dying of a heart attack at a tantra retreat.

On the plus side, it would be less humiliating than going

to A&E with a jade egg up me, on account of the fact that I'd be dead.

But what would they say to mum?

On the second night I walked through the door to the main room, and saw something I had been in too blind a panic to notice before: a table set up like an altar with flowers, eastern-looking statues and a plate full of condoms, sitting there like hors d'oeuvres.

Hippy Enya piped up on the speakers. The pain in my chest intensified.

'Does everybody have their blindfolds?' asked Jan.

We did.

We put them on and my chest hurt and my bowels felt like they were about to initiate a mass evacuation. All I could think of was the condoms.

With the blindfolds on, Jan invited us to move to the music.

I moved, but was still thinking of the condoms.

Then her soft, spacy voice told us that we could remove a layer of clothes if we wanted to.

What? This was only the second night! We couldn't be doing this on the second night. I thought that maybe some people might get naked on the last night – but not now! If we were doing this on the second night *what were we going to be doing for the rest of the week?*

The chest pain now felt like a steel vice on my heart.

This was awful.

Too much.

Really too much.

I didn't want to get undressed. No way.

But what if everyone else was naked and I was the only prude with her clothes on?

Pull yourself together, Marianne. In Germany they do this all the time! If you were there you'd be naked in a sauna and no big deal. You got naked for that art class. Don't be a loser.

I took off my T-shirt and moved my blindfold in the process. Through the gap at the bottom of my blindfold I could see that I was wearing an old beige-ish bra that had gone a blue-grey from being put in too many dark washes. One of the underwires had started to come out and was visible in the middle. I hadn't *Pussy*-fied it out of my wardrobe on account of only having three bras, but now I wished I had. And why hadn't I brought the fancy Greek underwear that was still sitting in that drawer, only worn to my romantic dinner for one? How on earth had I not thought to bring nice underwear to a tantra retreat? But when I'd read up on it, it had all been about boundaries! I didn't think we were going to be naked!

I couldn't be seen in this bra. My boobs were less embarrassing than this bra. I took it off and felt my boobs drop. I tried to look through the gap at the bottom of my blindfold at what the others were doing. I could see bare legs.

No, no, no.

Everyone was naked, weren't they?

Jan suggested in a soothing tone that we could now remove our blindfolds and begin to walk around the room and look each other up and down.

No, no, no! I didn't want to do this.

I didn't want to walk around topless with all these gross, pervy men in a room near a golf course in Sussex! I didn't want these men to see my boobs!

I started to walk.

And then I went blank.

The next thing I remember, I was putting my top back on again, and walking, shaking, up to my room.

My roommate looked just as shocked as I was.

'I don't know if I can stay the whole week,' I said.

'Me neither.'

'No, but really, I'm not just saying it – I don't think I can,' I repeated.

'Me neither.'

'Did you drive here?' I asked.

'No, I got the train.'

'Me too.'

'But we could call a cab to the station, if we had to,' she said.

'Yes.'

That night I lay in bed. Rigid. Awake. Petrified.

At some point I asked: 'Are you still awake?'

'Yes,' she said into the dark.

But we had nothing more to say. No comfort to offer each other.

I must have dozed a bit because I woke at dawn to a dimly lit room. My roommate was breathing heavily. I got up and went down to the kitchen. I took a mug from the shelf and topped it up with hot water from the giant silver urn.

'Good morning.' I looked up to see the religion teacher had walked in.

'Morning,' I replied.

'How are you doing?' she asked as she made tea.

'I don't think I can do this,' I blurted. 'I feel like I'm having a heart attack – like I have a pain in my chest, and . . . and yesterday, last night, I took my top off and I didn't want to but I did and now I feel sick that I walked around topless.'

Her chocolate eyes shined at me.

'You overstepped your boundaries. You dishonoured yourself by doing something you didn't want to do.'

'Yeah, but sometimes you have to make yourself do things

you don't want to do – surely? I just feel like I need to push myself otherwise I'd do nothing. Like I don't want to do my tax return, but I have to – don't we just have to do things we don't want to?'

'I don't think this is like a tax return.'

'Sorry, I know. That was a stupid thing to say.'

Her gaze stayed on my face, while mine darted from her face to the table.

'Lots of people kept their clothes on,' she said.

'Did they?'

'Yes. Didn't you see?'

I thought back, and she was right – I could picture quite a few people with their clothes still on.

Why didn't I think that I was allowed to do that?

'Jan keeps saying that we should never do anything we don't want to do,' the religion teacher said.

'Does she?'

'Yes, didn't you hear that?'

'I don't know.' I was so locked in my own head, beating myself up for being a prude and imagining how free everyone else was that actually I hadn't heard a lot of what she said.

'She said that we should push ourselves a bit, but never so much that it feels overwhelming.'

'Just being in that room feels overwhelming to me.'

'Well, don't do anything more then. Just being in the room is enough, and if that feels too much, take breaks.'

'I'm going to the loo constantly, I'm shitting all the time! Is that too much information?'

'It's OK.'

'I don't understand why, 'cause I've been too freaked out to eat anything, and yet I keep going to the loo. I actually don't know where it's coming from!'

'You're letting go of shit!' she smiled.

'I'm scared shitless!' I agreed.

I was usually too uptight for toilet humour, but this felt like a relief.

Others were coming in now to make tea and coffee, wearing yoga pants and shell-shocked expressions. Still, I was convinced that I was the most pathetic. Deep down these people had normal relationships and were OK, in ways that I wasn't.

'I don't understand what's wrong with me.'

Her big brown eyes kept looking at me.

'You just seem so cool with it all and so able to talk about your body and I've never talked about my body, and . . . and . . . "sex" stuff' – even saying the word 'sex' felt new and awkward in my mouth – 'and you just *can* . . . I dunno. Like on the first night when we did that exercise I thought you'd all think I was a prude if I didn't want to be touched, but I didn't want it. I didn't want anyone to touch me, and it's not because you aren't nice, I just didn't want it . . . I don't know you . . . and then when I touched you all I kept thinking was that I was doing it wrong . . . and my hands were sweaty and gross, and then I figured that you were all OK with all of this and I'm a freak 'cause I don't know what to do.'

She kept nodding empathetically as I spoke.

'It's taken a lot of work for me to get where I am.'

She explained that she had come from a religious background and very strict, much older parents. 'As a teenager, I thought that if I kissed a boy I'd go to hell,' she laughed. 'I'm laughing now, but I really thought that. I never saw any affection between my parents, who were quite Victorian, I suppose. My father was in the Army, a good man but a strict one . . . he didn't ever hug me. And my mother was not a happy woman. So I probably grew up with a fear around men, and a sense that sex was morally wrong.'

She paused, before continuing: 'I had a privileged child-hood, but it's been a long journey to dismantle what I learned about sex and relationships. I'm still working at it.'

'You're very brave.'

She smiled at me. 'Thank you. I'm just going to let that land.'

She closed her eyes and put her hands to her chest. She took a deep breath like she was smelling the ocean. She opened her eyes again and smiled. There was a silence as she kept looking at me and I kept looking at her and it all felt a bit too intense and my chest started to hurt again.

'I need to go to the loo,' I said.

And so it turned out the biggest lesson in my tantra week was the opposite of what I thought it would be – it wasn't about pushing myself, it was about going very easy on myself and saying 'no'.

After my morning chat, I was paired up with 'er, Jay', the man with the tufty bit of hair under his lip. He asked if he could stroke my face. 'No,' I said. Saying 'no' felt thrilling. The power! The control! Who knew I had that?

He nodded.

'Can I stroke your arm?'

I thought about it. I wanted to say yes, and so I did.

As he stroked my arm I got shivers. It felt good . . . too good. What was I doing standing in a room with a strange man stroking my arm?

'Stop,' I said. He looked at me kindly. I felt annoyed that I'd stopped it.

'Would you like a hug?' he asked.

I thought about it.

'Yes.'

He opened his arms and made a 'mmm' sound again as he gripped me, and I felt myself stiffen. I didn't like this. The arm stroke I'd liked, but this . . . no.

Old me would have just stayed there until he was finished – giving the man what he wanted – but this time I said 'goodbye', to signal the end of the encounter. He stepped back and I felt guilty. It felt wrong to reject him like that. I imagined I was disappointing him and hurting him and that he wished he'd partnered up with someone else – someone who would give him long, sexy hugs. Not this repressed Catholic.

'I'm sorry I said goodbye to you,' I said, when we were given time later to share how it had been for us.

'Why are you sorry?'

'I felt bad – like I was rejecting you.'

'I feel relieved when I hear a clear "no", because then I know that you're looking after yourself and I can relax.'

'Oh.'

'It makes me feel better about approaching you in later exercises because I know that you wouldn't do anything you didn't want to.'

'Oh. OK. I worried I'd hurt your feelings.'

He shook his head. 'It's good for me to hear "no", it's something I'm working on. A few years ago it would have triggered me into feeling unwanted, but now it doesn't.'

He had also done a fair amount of 'sexuality work' – everyone referred to it as 'work', which I thought was funny, and also, as the week went on, accurate.

His reaction was the exact opposite to the one I'd imagined. I wondered how often I'd done things I didn't want to in order to give someone something I thought they wanted, but which wasn't actually what they wanted, or maybe needed.

Jan asked us to notice how easy it was for us to say 'yes' or 'no'.

'Could you say "yes" when you really meant "yes"?' she asked. 'Could you say "yes" without shame or judgement? Or do you feel so scared of the "yes" your body was saying that you shut down and run out of the room?' She continued to probe: 'How easy was it to say "no" when you didn't like a touch? Did you find yourself saying "no" because you were too scared to say "yes"?'

I thought about it. I'd said 'yes' to the hug, and then 'no' when it didn't feel good. And I had actually wanted to keep saying 'yes' to the arm stroking but stopped it because I was ashamed of it feeling good. Good girls shouldn't enjoy having their arms stroked by strangers in function rooms in Sussex.

I noticed how much I was policing myself. Showing – or even feeling – any pleasure felt dirty and wrong, just as it had when I tried to love my own body at home.

Both 'yes' and 'no' brought problems. I worried my 'no' would upset people, that my 'yes' would get me into situations I couldn't get out of. In my usual life, I would have said nothing at all, I would have been silent and frozen, expecting people to be mind-readers and resenting them when they weren't.

Jan gave us examples of different kinds of 'yes' and 'no', revealing just how fraught these seemingly simple words were. First, we say 'yes' when we mean 'no' because we think it will make people like us. I had done that. Not so much with sex but with everything else. (Yeah, sure I'll feed your cats, meet you miles away from where I live, yeah, sure . . .) We say 'yes' to avoid difficult conversations or hurting other people's feelings. We say 'yes' to avoid conflict. To be seen as nice or good people.

Story of my life.

Jan asked if we sometimes said 'yes' because we hope we'll get something in return.

Hmm. Yes.

Did we sometimes say 'yes' instead of 'no' because we think it's the kind thing to do?

Oh my god, yes. Normally I would have stayed in that uncomfortable hug for as long as er-Jay had wanted because it would have felt unkind to step away. But Jan explained that doing things to be kind is often not kind.

'Other people's feelings are their business,' Jan told us. 'It's not your responsibility to manage them.' What's more, she explained, difficult feelings can be very valuable if they help someone face something they've been avoiding. Also, saying 'no' when you mean 'no' is a kindness to the other person, who can relax knowing that you are speaking the truth.

And there is a great cost to us saying 'yes' when we want to say 'no'.

Jan explained: 'When we say "yes" to things we don't want to, we are likely to numb out so that we don't have to endure feelings of having betrayed ourselves. We give ourselves away in exchange for love and approval.' Oh god.

We find 'no' both hard to say and to hear because as children a 'no' can be terrifying. We need love for survival and a 'no' can be a sign that we have displeased our parents and might be rejected. This can feel life-threatening. Even as adults we can still associate the word 'no' with the sense that we are bad in some way, and that people will stop loving us.

And because so many of us are shy of using it, it means that we don't get to hear it much, which makes it all the more shocking when we do. Hearing and saying 'no' is a muscle we need to build.

'It's not a rejection if somebody doesn't want to be with you – it's just information,' she said. I wasn't sure about that. It sure felt like a rejection. And a criticism. And a confirmation of everything I knew to be wrong about myself. 'When you say "no" when you mean "no" you are giving someone the gift of honesty.'

She explained that it was not kind to be with someone if you didn't want to be with them, because you were holding them back from being with someone who would want to be with them. 'Nobody wants to be with someone who does not want to be with them,' she said. It sounded so obvious as she said it.

Jan talked about how we might say 'no' to something because we fear that by saying 'yes' we are signing up to something more. So we say 'no' to having a coffee with someone because we think that if we say 'yes', they will want to meet for dinner, and if we meet for dinner we'll have to have sex. And if we have sex we'll end up in a relationship and then we'll probably get married. So you say 'no' to the coffee because you don't want to marry this person.

The room laughed. I had done this.

'You can change your mind, at any point,' she explained. 'A "yes" is a "yes" just in this moment. It is not a "yes" to everything.' I realized that's how I operated. It was easier to say 'no' – or rather completely avoid – interactions instead of getting caught up in potentially hurting people's feelings later down the line and having difficult conversations.

This was a revelation: this idea that I didn't have to do anything I didn't want to do. I didn't have to please others, or do what I thought was expected. It took a while to sink in.

I thought it was selfish to only do what I wanted to do. But Jan was saying it wasn't selfish. It was actually the best thing for everybody.

I kept repeating it in my head, like a mantra. 'I don't have to do anything I don't want to do. I don't have to do anything I don't want to do . . .'

———

As I started to lean into this idea, I started to relax. Well, a bit. The shitting and sweating continued, but there were some points in the following days when I didn't have chest pains.

After every exercise each person was invited to say how it had been for them. People spoke with great detail and honesty. I said 'fine' a lot. I could see how often I stayed silent for fear of saying something that would hurt others. Learning to say things out loud was a challenge, but whatever I voiced was met with kindness. It was a revelation.

As Hawaiian Santa put it, we were changing our lives one mortifying sentence at a time.

Gradually, I started to relax. Instead of feeling guarded with others, I felt joy. And instead of feeling tired in their company, I felt revived. I wondered if the reason I felt so tired with people was because I was usually putting on an act, trying to be whatever that other person wanted me to be. It was something I did automatically. I hadn't even known I was doing it till now.

In the breaks we ran to the nearby beach and swam in the cold twinkling sea, laughing and splashing like children. In the evenings we'd pile on the sofas like puppies, giggling and hugging each other. It felt so natural. One evening I sat next to one of the necklace-wearers, who had announced he was 'available for hugs' and who had given me the creeps at first. His neediness had repelled me. Now I leaned my head on his shoulder as we chatted.

'Thank you for touching me,' he said.

Nobody had ever said that to me before.

'In my normal life the only time I get touched is at the hair-dressers . . . And I'm running out of hair to cut.' He rubbed his almost bald skull and smiled at the joke but felt sad.

'Don't you hug your friends?' I asked.

'Guys don't really do that in Ipswich,' he said.

I felt grateful to be a woman who could hug her friends.

We talked about how with friends, physical contact was limited to pecks on the cheek or quick hugs, and with the opposite sex all contact had to be a prelude to sex. But here it wasn't like that. There was an innocence to touch that didn't ever have to lead to anything more. It was a relief to be close to others without any feeling of pressure. Without the feeling that every contact was somehow leading to something or being sexualized. I hadn't realized how much I was starving for touch, my body soaked it up like a dry sponge.

As the days passed, I was able to let go of my fear that all the men in the group were gropy, predatory weirdos – because they weren't. Well, apart from the elephant T-shirt guy. He claimed to be able to have sex telepathically with people in India but on day three he had a plumbing emergency and had to leave early.

On the last two days we were each to have an 'initiation ceremony', in which we were to be welcomed into our sexuality in a way that we never were as teenagers. We were asked to line up and pick people we wanted to 'serve us'. Then we stood in line and waited to be picked.

I panicked. The certainty of rejection was too much.

'Nobody is going to pick me!' I cried, loud enough so that the room of fifty people turned to look at me.

I was right back to being a kid at my first disco, terrified I would not be asked to dance . . . I realized that I carried that feeling with me every day. I was not the girl – woman – that boys – men – asked to dance. I was not one of the pretty blonde girls called Sarah, I was a chubby-chopped ginger who—

'I'll pick you!' Hawaiian Santa said. Then 'er, Jay' with the hair-tuft said he would too and then several more, and the relief was vast, but before I could enjoy it it was my turn to pick who would serve me, and that was almost as excruciating. I didn't want men to know that I fancied them. I avoided the hot guy – obviously – and chose two men and a woman who made me feel safe: Hawaiian Santa, 'er, Jay' and Anna the religion teacher.

When the time came to serve others, I worried I would not be good enough, that I would do something wrong.

'You can't do anything wrong,' Hawaiian Santa said when it was his turn. 'Do what you want to do, and no more.' It was a gift.

And then it was time for my initiation. Before it began we were asked to tell the other three where and how we wanted to be touched. I still felt shy of this but as I looked at their three pairs of kind eyes, I also felt safe.

By this point in the week some people had progressed to full stages of undress during the touching. We were constantly told not to look at what other people were doing, only to stay present with ourselves and the people we were with, but occasionally I'd catch a glimpse of flesh.

'I'm going to keep my clothes on,' I said.

They nodded.

'No touching my boobs or – or – um – genitals.'

They nodded again and smiled.

'OK. That's it.'

'Do you like touch to be light or firm?' Anna asked.

I didn't know what I liked.

'Light, maybe. But not tickly light – um, I dunno.'

'It's OK, tell us if there's anything you don't like,' said Santa.

'OK.'

I lay on the mattress and these three adult faces looked down at me, smiling, smiling, smiling.

I had a lump in my throat and the chest pain was starting again.

'I'm scared,' I said, big fat tears streaming down my cheeks.

'You'll be OK, we're here,' said Anna, squeezing my arm.

Jan started talking on her mic, instructing those of us who were being initiated to start breathing in a precise way. With each breath, we had to tilt our pelvis up off the ground. As we breathed out, we were to let the base of our spine thump down into the mattress.

While we were doing this we were to look, non-stop, into the eyes of one of our servers. I looked into Anna's eyes and I felt her strength and her love and her sisterhood. I had no idea how long this breathing lasted for but at some point things started to feel a bit trippy and then my servers started to touch me.

I closed my eyes and felt gentle sweeping strokes begin up my arms and down my legs and my whole body. I felt self-conscious.

It felt selfish to just be lying here without doing anything for anyone. I should be doing something for them. This one-way street wasn't right. I worried that it was boring for them that I was keeping all my clothes on.

I worried I should be feeling more. I wasn't feeling anything.

Then I felt a hand on my thigh.

I bet they're thinking it's too big . . .

Stop it. Be polite, Marianne. Breathe. Smile. You should smile, be grateful.

Jan had clearly said that we could say stop at any time, but that we should not have conversations . . . or issue requests.

This was a chance to surrender into love. But should I whisper 'thank you' and tell them that they didn't have to be here if they didn't want to, they could go and make a cup of tea if they were bored?

And should I be feeling more now? Moaning? Making a show of it? Why wasn't I feeling more?

I opened my eyes and Anna had been replaced by a goddess whose dark blue, kind eyes were looking in mine – willing me on, it felt like, willing me to surrender – and I looked at the two men who seemed genuinely enraptured by their job of stroking my fully-clothed calves.

I closed my eyes and worried again that this was boring for them. If they found another group they'd be able to get naked and have a much more exciting time. They'd be all orgasmic and—

I bet they think you're a prude, I bet they think you're—

Stop it, Marianne. Stop it, stop it, stop it, breathe, breathe, breathe . . .

I thought of Jan's words, or somebody's words: 'To feel more you have to breathe more.'

Breathe, breathe, breathe . . .

I felt my shoulders drop, and then someone took my hand and held it firmly. I opened my eyes and saw it was Hawaiian Santa. Something in me gave way and now I was crying, crying at the feeling of safety that I so rarely felt with other people. Crying at the love I could feel with every touch.

'Touch touches more than your skin,' Jan had said earlier. 'It touches the feelings stored in our bodies, it touches memories of the times we have and have not been touched. It touches all the emotions that are stored in our bodies.'

I was crying for the lack of closeness I'd had in my life, how I'd stayed away from physical touch for fear of getting hurt or smothered, for fear of being rejected and laughed at . . . for fear of not being good enough. I was suddenly awash with grief about how much I had cut myself off from love.

I had an image of my life being lived deep underground in a damp basement, away from everyone. I felt my heart would break with the sadness and as I sobbed and my hand kept being held, I opened my eyes and saw three pairs of eyes looking at me with love, love, love, love . . .

I looked at Santa and 'er, Jay', trusting them completely. These beautiful, kind men.

Jan's voice came over the microphone, her voice calm, devotional, serene. 'Don't cut off pleasure, say yes to it all.'

As I'd seen in my self-love month, I had cut off from pleasure, because pleasure felt wrong and dirty and like something I didn't deserve. I'd felt I didn't deserve this love and attention . . . but *why* didn't I? And what was wrong with pleasure? This was beautiful and pure and innocent.

I felt a pang in my chest that reminded me of the feeling I used to get when I looked at my A-ha poster as a young girl. The longing. Deep longing.

The feathery strokes felt like they were getting faster, six hands sweeping over me, and I dropped into another place, outside normal time and space. I surrendered, I trusted, I let go. And it felt divine . . .

And then it was over.

My glimpse of heaven.

6

Old Friends

'Did you take your clothes off?' Rachel asked.

'No! Well, kind of, at the beginning, and then I felt crap and put them back on.'

'Did you snog anyone?'

'Kind of, but it wasn't really like that—'

'With tongues?'

'Yes . . . kind of.'

'Why do you keep saying "kind of"?'

'I don't know, it's just it wasn't really like that—'

'Did you snog a woman?'

'No.'

'And you didn't shag anyone?'

'No.'

'And were other people shagging?'

'I don't know.'

'What do you mean you don't know?'

'I mean I don't know – they tell you to just focus on yourself . . . not to look at others . . .'

'But do you think they were?'

'Honestly, I don't know. I don't think so. What news on egg freezing?' I asked, to change the subject.

She lifted up her T-shirt and I saw the bruises on her tummy.

'From the hormone injections. I can't be arsed to talk about it.'

'OK.'

'So if you didn't shag anyone what were you doing?'

I found it hard to put into words. The idea of fifty strangers touching each other and practising saying 'yes' and 'no' sounded strange in the normal world, and yet when we were there it was so beautiful.

Since I'd come home, I kept replaying the final evening of the workshop like it was a movie. It had been a stormy night and we danced with the wind under the stars. I'd felt alive and sexy and innocent and free, one with the trees and the stars and dark night sky . . . one with everyone around me.

It was a moment of perfect happiness.

There was no judgement of men's necklaces or facial hair, no fear of other people's judgement towards me – there was just love. I was dancing in love and it felt divine, mystical almost.

I'd never felt anything like it before.

Back home, I kept dancing. I had no interest in watching people killing each other on Netflix or drinking wine, instead I spent the evenings dancing in my living room, enjoying the feeling of my body moving. If Daisy was home she'd join me, or we'd go to Ecstatic Dance.

I went for slow walks where I kept stopping to gaze at the cotton-ball clouds and felt turned on by trees. I videoed them dancing in the wind, shimmying in the breeze, the little flirts. I felt the wind blowing on my skin and it felt like being kissed. My body hummed with life. Colours seemed brighter.

I felt almost porous, as if I was connected to everything and everyone around me. This, according to Jan, was what happens when your sexual energy is allowed to flow instead of being suppressed. We feel more awake and energetic, we see the beauty in everything and feel the sensation of everything.

I kept thinking of my initiation and how my body had felt being touched and loved and stroked by three people for two hours. I'd never experienced anything like that before. How many of us had experienced this? Being touched without any expectation of reciprocating? Being touched without it ever having to lead to anything else?

The week of tantra had helped me to thaw. To wake up.

But what now?

Life outside tantra was not nearly touch-y enough. I yearned to spend a good ten minutes looking into the eyes of the guy in the organic shop and giving him a good breathing-in-and-out 'mmm'-hug, but I sensed he wouldn't have been OK with that. Jan had told us that every moment of the day we could be in touch with our sexual energy, whether we were with someone or not.

'Embody your sexual woman at the supermarket!' she said. 'Take a deep breath and smell the fruit and vegetables and allow yourself to be turned on by them.' What? Turned on by a tomato? Turns out the tomatoes didn't do it for me – but aubergines glistening under the lights could get me going.

I tried Pant-Free Friday again, this time with flowing yoga trousers instead of jeans. It felt nice.

That night I made a roast vegetable salad. I ate alone by candlelight, as I had done during *Pussy*. This time it didn't feel awkward or sad, it felt beautiful. Everything felt beautiful. Afterwards I showered and enjoyed the smell of the Mysore soap I'd bought in the local hippy shop that was run by a Sufi mother and son. I enjoyed the feeling of the soap touching my body. This time it didn't feel wrong to feel my body and to enjoy those feelings. It felt entirely natural.

When I got out of the shower I looked into the full-length

mirror. For perhaps the first time in my life, I allowed myself to feel beautiful.

It helped that my week of eating vegetables and pooing constantly meant I'd lost five pounds. They should put that in the brochure. Sexual healing and weight loss. But it was far more than weight loss. Something deeper had changed in me. I felt different.

People were noticing it.

Daisy told me I looked very 'embodied'.

'What does that mean?' I asked.

'You are very in your body.' This was a phrase I'd heard people use during the tantra week and I didn't understand it. Of course I was in my body, where else would I be?

'Aren't I always in my body?' I asked Daisy.

'I think sometimes you are very in your head,' she said.

That was true.

Pussy had shown me how cut off I was from my body and, according to Daisy, most of us were. In the West we live in a very 'heady' place – where our body is just this thing that carries our head around and which we criticize for not looking right. Our poor bodies . . .

Now I was enjoying this body of mine. Not just how it looked, but how it felt. And I had *so much* energy – I was at once wide awake and able to sleep deeply, my body felt soft, my mind calm, and everything looked beautiful. I craved wearing colours instead of my usual greys.

The Greek Skyped.

'You're shining,' he said.

I didn't tell him why. I'd discovered that I couldn't explain it in a way that let people really get it. They wanted to hear the juicy bits and I felt irritated by this limited view of sex, as something naughty. The week had been rich and deep and truly beautiful, but I didn't know how to explain that without sounding like a spiritual Mills & Boon. 'It felt like being in a different world!' I wanted to say. 'I fell in love with everyone! I felt more human and free and at ease with myself than I'd ever felt before! Touch felt natural and beautiful and not at all icky or pervy.' It sounded strange, so I soon learned to keep quiet.

'So did you have an orgy then?' my sister asked as we watched *Strictly*.

'No,' I said.

She didn't ask any more.

I told mum I had been on a 'communication course'.

'What kind of communication?'

'I don't want to talk about it.'

By the time I went to Sarah's my erotic adventures felt like a dream, and now I had woken up.

'Ella has nits.'

We were at the breakfast bar in her new house in Kent. Beyond glass doors was a muddy garden with a trampoline by a falling-down fence. There were toys and plates everywhere and the radio in the kitchen was competing with the cartoons Ella was watching in the living room next door.

'We got an email from the school. Could you take a look to see if I have them too? I've got one of those little combs.'

We moved to the window and I examined her scalp.

'I can't see anything.'

'Can you comb through anyway, just in case?'

'Yeah, of course.'

She passed me a tiny metal comb.

'This is a proper grown-up house!' I said, looking around. My rented flat was the size of her kitchen.

'Yeah, there's still lots to do, but—'

'There's no rush,' I said. 'What are the new neighbours like?'

She rolled her eyes. '*Grand Designs* houses and smiles that don't meet their eyes. The other day I dropped Ella off for a playdate and I asked the woman if I should take my shoes off, and she said, "Don't worry, you won't be staying".'

'Bloody hell.'

'Oh, yeah, she was really something.'

'Your hair is so shiny,' I said, moving the comb through, enjoying the intimacy of combing her hair and smelling her shampoo.

'I look like a badger, I can't afford to get the greys done.'

'Apparently grey is popular now – some woman in *Vogue* wrote about letting hers go completely natural. How's Ella?'

'She's OK. We had to take her in a couple of nights ago because she had problems breathing but they got it sorted.'

'God, that's scary.'

Sarah shrugged. She had been in hospital so many times since Ella was born prematurely.

It was a cliché to say I didn't know how she did it, but I didn't know how she did it.

She asked about the tantra and I felt embarrassed to talk about it. She was in hospital with Ella while I was walking around with my top off and learning to say 'yes' and 'no'. She looked horrified when I told her there were couples there.

'Married couples?'

'Yeah.'

Her phone beeped. She checked it. 'Shit.'

'What is it?'

'It's going to cost nine hundred pounds to get the car fixed.'

'Shit.'

'It wasn't even my fault.'

'That's annoying.'

'Fuck.'

'Look, at least you weren't badly hurt – is your back better?'

'It's OK. I'm going to a chiropractor which costs a fucking fortune, and the roof is leaking which is going to cost another God knows how much.'

I got the feeling I increasingly had around friends – that they were living proper, grown-up lives with grown-up responsibilities, while I was in a perpetual state of adolescence.

After lunch, we went to the park.

Sarah chatted to other mums and I smiled and nodded my way through chat about playdates and the gossip of someone losing it on the class WhatsApp group. I felt myself receding. The swings creaked under a concrete sky. Women stood around in green parkas and expensive trainers.

'Do you have kids?' one asked.

'No . . . I don't,' I said and smiled, to soften the 'no'. I always felt uncomfortable with that 'no'. It sounded so stark. So abrupt. Like I was a heartless cow who wanted to eat children instead of give birth to them. I wanted to back it up with 'I really like kids,' to assure her that I was not a cold-hearted bitch, followed by 'I just never felt the need to have my own . . .' – but then I worried that last bit would in some way seem like a criticism of her choices.

'Lucky you!' she smiled. She was nice.

I wondered if she was imagining a sad story for me, one in which I never met the right guy and was now trying to pretend that I liked my independence. 'Poor thing' she was probably thinking.

But maybe that was all in my head. This woman probably wasn't thinking about me at all, she was too busy trying to stop her son mount a campaign to get a little girl off the swing.

'Oscar, leave her – I said leave her! Wait your turn – or go on the slide instead. Sorry,' she said, turning to me again. 'As soon as she's off the swing, he won't be interested.'

I watched as Oscar stomped through those wood chip things to a red slide and eyed up two bigger boys sitting at the top of it. He wasn't going to pester them to get off.

'Marianne's just been at a tantra week,' said Sarah.

The woman didn't know how to arrange her face in response to this sentence.

'Wow! Lucky you!' she said again. She really was nice.

'Ha! Yeah, it was interesting,' I tried to be jokey.

'I can't even remember what sex is, it's all cobwebs down there . . .' She said with a tired smile. I smiled back an equally tired smile.

We were both tired of our roles – her as a knackered mum looking forward to wine o'clock, and me as the crazy single girl going off to sex weeks – but we didn't know how to get beyond them.

I made my excuses so that I would be on time to meet Daisy.

'What are you up to now?' asked Sarah.

'It's Ecstatic Dance, remember that hippy dancing thing I went to before?'

'Like Rainbow Rhythms?' she asked.

'That's the one,' I said.

'Our lives are so different,' Sarah said, kissing me on the cheek.

It felt like a judgement.

Nobody teaches you how to navigate friendships. They are supposed to happen effortlessly, and for a good chunk of my life they did. I might not have found relationships with men easy but I had been blessed with friends.

Since my friends started having children and moving out of London, things had, inevitably, changed. We used to run to the same schedule – manic work and manic after-work drinking. Even when they got married, we stayed largely the same. But now our lives were, as Sarah pointed out, so different.

They were at the school gates, I was semi-naked in a hall with strangers. They had jobs and houses and partners and children, I was flirting with courgettes.

They didn't have a spare second. I had nothing but spare seconds.

My life felt selfish and stupid compared to theirs – ridiculous, almost. From the minute they woke up, they were looking after someone else. I had only myself to think about. My news and worries felt petty and insignificant, while they were keeping sick children alive, and so, increasingly, I kept quiet.

When people asked how I was, I'd quickly turn it back, asking instead about their spouses, roof extensions, babies' sleeping habits. My life felt less real than theirs. When I did talk, I felt it was my job to be entertaining, to make light of my life, like a single court jester.

'Do you find it hard to be around friends with kids?' I'd asked Rachel on the phone later.

'Yeah, I guess. I get bored of schlepping to them because they don't want to get a babysitter, or having them cancel at the last minute because someone's got a puking thing. Half the time I think they just can't be arsed.'

'Yeah, maybe.'

'It pisses me off. If you have a family, you have an inbuilt social life – if I don't make plans to see people, I'll be at home on my own.'

'I like being home on my own,' I said.

'I don't,' she replied. 'And I'm fed up with always going to their houses – why is my life meant to fit in around theirs? I mean, I'm OK with it most of the time, but not all the time. Nobody comes to me any more.'

I liked going to my friends' houses and being cooked for. I liked using Sarah's bath and loved it when she left me pillow spray and an eye mask in her spare room.

I asked Daisy the same question later. 'Do you feel different to your friends with kids?'

'Not really,' she said. 'I know a couple of people with kids but we're not really close, so it's not a thing. I, um . . . I don't really have the friendships that you do – I always found guys easier.'

This time it was my turn to say: 'Our lives are so different.'

Our lives were changing, and with them our friendships. But we didn't seem to have the language to talk about it. In relationships, we had the big *'What is this?'* conversations. With friendships, we didn't. We just bumbled along and pretended everything was OK. I especially did this because I'd spent my life running from conflict and difficult conversations. Running away from difficult conversations was often the only exercise I got.

As friends were absorbed in work and family life, I spent more and more time corresponding with strangers on the internet, people who got in touch after reading my writing. I liked these kinds of connections because they were usually telling me how great I was. And it wasn't just me – I'd been reading about something called 'parasocial' relationships, which are the one-sided relationships we develop with people we will never know, people on television, on Instagram. It seemed that we were losing the patience and commitment to keep our real-life friendships alive over long working hours,

family routines and geographical distance. Sometimes friendships felt more like an admin task than a joy.

According to headlines, we were living in the loneliest time
ever in human existence. Forty-one per cent of British people
said that the TV or a pet was their main source of company. The situation was so extreme that Former US Surgeon
General Vivek Murthy had said, 'During my years caring for
patients, the most common pathology I saw was not heart
disease or diabetes. It was loneliness.'

Having good friends, on the other hand, has been shown
to boost the immune system and our ability to deal with
chronic pain. It also makes us happier, with studies showing that when somebody claims to have five or more friends,
they are 60 per cent more likely to say that they are very
happy.

I read an article about friendship in which a psychologist
argued that there's no such thing as being too busy to meet
people. If you spent four hours a night watching Netflix but
you didn't make time for your friends, you had your priorities
wrong. Which was true to a point . . . but energy and geog-
raphy were also massive factors. But maybe these were just
excuses.

It was time to make more effort to prioritize and nurture
my friendships.

I ordered several books about friendship, including Dr
Murthy's book *Together*, *The Meaning of Friendship* by Mark
Vernon and *Friendship* by A. C. Grayling, and put them on the
side of my bed, on top of *Pussy* and my single books.

My therapist had other ideas.

'Maybe it's time to make some new friends,' she suggested.

'I love my friends.'

'I'm not suggesting you drop your old friendships, but it might be helpful to see people living different kinds of lives.'

'Maybe,' I said. 'But I don't want to live a different life, I want to be normal.'

She made a face that looked like she'd smelled something bad. 'Why on earth would you want that?' she asked.

I laughed. 'Because not being normal is lonely.'

'I imagine your friends have experienced great loneliness looking after their children,' she said.

I remembered mum talking about how lonely it was when I was a baby and she'd moved to England and knew nobody but dad who was at work all the time.

'What are you thinking?' the therapist asked me.

'Nothing,' I said.

I told her about the tantra retreat.

'Sounds wonderful,' she said. 'Will you do more?'

'There are more workshops, but I don't know – it's expensive and I was thinking that I should probably put more energy into my friends, be there for them more. They have so much going on, and I could help them more than I do.'

'That's an admirable sentiment,' she replied, 'but you also have your own life to live.'

7

New Friends

I was trying to read *The Meaning of Friendship* by Mark Vernon but I was finding it hard to concentrate. The road outside was being dug up, so every day I sat at my desk to the sound of drilling. It was shaping up to be a warm summer and my flat was heating up like a greenhouse.

And so, when Daisy asked me if I wanted to go to a festival – something I'd spent my whole adult life saying no to – I said yes. It was in Devon and the deal was that if I didn't like it, Daisy would drive me to the station, no questions asked. I packed my suitcase again.

We listened to Alanis Morrisette and the Cranberries on the way there. We stopped off at a service station and I bought M&S chocolate bites for the tent. I had eaten half of them by the time we got there, while Daisy nibbled on nuts.

We turned down a dirt track. Signs for the festival, hand-painted on large pieces of board, told us we were on the right track. A car turned in behind us, a battered campervan driven by a man with long hair and a woman and child next to him. A long-haired man with a hi-vis vest over a bare brown chest directed us to our parking spot.

Daisy jumped straight out and started to unpack the car. She'd brought a large fold-down trolley for us to load the tent, bags of food, sleeping bags and fairy lights onto and tied it all in with bungee cords. She had a whole system, born of years of festival-going.

While we hauled our stuff down a grassy hill, I felt embarrassed by my wheelie Samsonite. Everyone around me was carefree hippy, with battered rucksacks and wheelbarrows full of gear.

Everyone we passed grinned and said hello. They just looked so happy to be in a field. So happy to be alive. It was unnerving. When Daisy's trolley toppled over, a man appeared from nowhere to help her get it back up. They walked together for a while. Of course he fancied Daisy. Everyone fancied Daisy. I felt invisible.

We arrived at a giant field of tents, spanning from one-man plastic numbers to enormous bell tents connected to other tents via porches.

'What about over there?' Daisy was saying, pointing at a spot under a tree. I had never put up a tent before and felt embarrassed by this as well. Fortunately she was a pro and only needed help with the pins, which I managed.

Once she'd wrapped fairy lights around the tent and filled it with blow-up mattresses and sheepskins, she declared, 'The tantric temple is open!' She was in her element, having grown up going to festivals with her mother. I was not in my element, because I had grown up going to swimming lessons in Camberley Leisure Centre and eating sandwiches on the beach in Kerry.

As we walked towards the main area of the festival to get some food, the sun was setting in a haze of ice-cream pinks and purples over the tops of tents nestled in the hills of Devon. Children with painted faces and butterfly wings were running around together, adults in technicolour outfits smiling and hugging. They had bright eyes and clear skin, piercings and dyed hair. They all looked like they bathed in a river.

It was idyllic. A paradise. And I hated it.

I might have felt like an alien in the park with the mums, but I felt like an alien here too.

I woke up to the sound of rain on my tent. I had been cold most of the night. My throat felt sore. The ground hard underneath my back, my air mattress no longer had air in it.

This was why I didn't do festivals.

I lay like a corpse looking at the rain splatting on the pink tent top and then over at Daisy, who was still asleep.

You're going to get sick. You shouldn't have come. Now you're trapped in a field in the middle of nowhere in the rain . . .

I unzipped my sleeping bag and rummaged for my wash bag. I fought with the zip that was our front door; it kept getting stuck.

Once I got out, I straightened up in the drizzle and felt a pit of depression as I looked at the sea of tents under a damp sky.

I made my way to the compost toilets.

I sat on the loo reading the flyers that were nailed to the inside of the wooden toilet door: 'Immersive coffin experience,' read one. 'For the coffin-curious – rest a while in a hand-woven coffin and let beautiful readings on life, death and impermanence wash over you. Booking essential.'

Another one promised to show you how to 'Emancipate Yourself from Mental Slavery Through the Gift of the Breath.'

I left and pulled out my bulging washbag.

A sleepy-looking Jesus with a bare chest wandered over to the sink plonked in the middle of grass to wash out an enamel cup. He was vegan. I could tell just by looking at him. He splashed his face with water and swirled some around in his mouth.

His beauty regime complete.

My Max White Colgate toothpaste felt wrong here. I bet everyone here used that aloe vera stuff you get in health food stores. Or baking soda. Or did that oil-swilling thing. I splashed water on my puffy face and went back to the tent and fought with the zip again.

Daisy was still asleep so I went in search of breakfast, walking past people doing yoga in the drizzle to get in line at a food tent, behind a woman wearing a long sequinned skirt and fluffy hoodie.

I'd ordered a load of random stuff on Amazon before coming – a headlight, a metal straw and something called a spork. Why didn't it occur to me to buy a waterproof jacket?

I felt a tap on my shoulder and turned around to see Daisy.

'Do you want anything?' I asked her.

'Green tea and before you say anything, the weather is going to clear. It says on my app.'

'OK,' I said, in my 'it's not OK' voice. I hated myself for it. The weather wasn't her fault. 'I just saw one of your friends and she said there have been thefts and that we should be careful,' I said.

'OK.'

'I didn't think hippies would have anything to steal.'

'You'd be surprised. The pashminas and bell tents are worth a bomb,' said Daisy. I couldn't tell if she was joking.

We had a vegetarian breakfast sitting on rugs around a low table. My bad mood brewed. I didn't want to be sitting on damp ground eating baked beans in a circus tent. I just didn't.

We walked to a huge notice board with the schedules for different workshops in different tents. Lucid Dreaming. Laughter Yoga. Trauma Release. Energy Cleansing with Stones. Mandala Making.

It was overwhelming. A spiritual Butlins.

'I've landed but I haven't arrived,' a woman behind me was saying.

Her friend agreed. 'I'm about half an inch here and half an inch above the ground. My adult wants to stay here and my child wants to go to Shamanic Trance Dance.'

'Do you want to go to Shamanic Trance Dance?' asked Daisy.

'No,' I said automatically even though I didn't know what it was.

'Or there's a flirting workshop, that sounds fun.'

'It sounds horrific,' I replied. But as I caught myself slipping further into this passive-aggressive sulk, I thought, No, Marianne, say it. Say the truth.

'Sorry – I'm in a bad mood, and I don't want to do any of the workshops or be around people. Do you mind if I do my own thing today?'

'Of course, love!' Daisy smiled. 'Good on you for stating your needs,' she said. Like it was no big deal. 'I'm going to do some yoga in the women's tent. I'll see you later.'

As she walked away I felt a bit confused by the lack of drama. Was it really that easy? I didn't have to do things I didn't want to do? And that was OK? I didn't have to pretend to be nice? Or happy? I could be a miserable cow and that was totally accepted?

I wondered if other friends would be this gracious about my request to do my own thing. I wondered whether, if Daisy had asked the same of me, I would be OK with it? Or would I have felt rejected?

I thought of the yeses and nos we'd learned at tantra, and my roommate being shocked by her friend who'd decided she didn't want to go to the cinema.

I made my way back to the tent to lie down, walking past

a naked man with a pot belly and a willy ring. I looked at my phone. It was II a.m.

I fell asleep for an hour or so, and when I woke up the sun was coming through the tent. I felt guilty about leaving Daisy. A good friend would have stayed with her. A good friend would not be in a mood. I rummaged through my bag to find my copy of *The Meaning of Friendship*. I still hadn't got past the first few pages. I would try again. The tent was heating up so I'd find a tree to sit under and read. On my own.

I unzipped the tent and found myself face to face with a man crouched outside his tent, cooking eggs on a stove.

'Hello!' he said. 'Would you like some tea? I'm just making breakfast.'

We chatted and he told me he was a builder. He used to be a punk and now he was a Buddhist. His name was Jim. He was wearing shoes that looked like they were made out of rope. He explained that they were some barefoot technology thing and that he wore them all year around – even in the snow in Manchester.

A woman with bright pink dreads walked past our tent – she seemed to know Jim. She talked about a vortex healing session she'd gone to the day before and was still 'processing'. Jim said he had booked in to do a sweat-lodge ceremony in the afternoon. He told us he'd done them before as part of an ayahuasca ceremony.

'Where did you do the ayahuasca?' I asked.

'Essex.'

I laughed. 'I thought you were going to say Peru or something.'

'No, it was in a community centre in Grays.'

'How was it?'

'Messy. They'd told us to wear white, which I did, but then

I puked and shat myself and I didn't have a change of clothes for the train home.'

I didn't know what to say.

'I figured it was a lesson in letting go of my vanity,' he shrugged.

If I wanted an unconventional world with people who didn't fit into the marriage, kids and renovating your kitchen set, I had found it. Suddenly, more than anything, I wanted to be at home doing my accounts.

After leaving Jim, I wandered around and found myself in an area with two domed saunas, a chill out tent and a garden with a fire in the middle. Everyone was naked. One woman was doing a naked downward dog, her small boobs like fried eggs. Another woman was being beaten with birch leaves by a skinny man with a nose ring.

They all had the bodies of people who believed that eating sugar is self-harming. I wished I was a stone lighter. I wished I'd gone on a diet before coming. I wished I didn't drink as much as I did or like chocolate, or carbs . . .

Stop it, Marianne! Stop it!

How long was this going to go on for, this constant scrutiny of the body? Seriously. Enough. Once and for all, enough.

I went to the changing dome, took off all my clothes and walked my naked non-yoga body into the open air, doing my best to pretend that this was totally normal for me.

Nobody seemed to notice.

I went to the sauna, opened the small rickety door and stooped to get in, worrying what my bum would look like at that angle, and then telling myself off for worrying.

And then, sweating in the darkness, I made a decision. For this week I would not care what I looked like and I would not

care about who did or didn't fancy me. I would not do things
I didn't want to do in order to be nice and make Daisy happy,
and I would not put on a big smile if I was in a bad mood.
But whatever happened, I would stay.

When it got too hot I went out and stood under a cold
shower rigged up by a tree. It was like ice. I was still worried
about the size of my arse but this time I laughed at myself.
So your arse is big. So what? Some guy you don't know might
look at you and think your arse is big. And?

I was greeted with friendly naked smiles, but for the first
time in my life I did not smile back. All my life I'd faked
smiles, done my best to be liked, to be 'nice', to keep my bad
moods to the confines of my bedroom. But fuck it!

It felt liberating not to care about the people around me.
Not to care about what they were thinking about me. Or
whether I was attractive to them or likeable. It was a relief
not to try to be funny or nice or good-looking. I could see
how much I spent my normal life trying to win people over,
trying to win a likeability contest. How fake it was. I caught
sight of a guy with washboard abs and two nipple rings.

Nipple rings. Why did people have them?

I went back into the black silent heat of the sauna and
thought about what a show-off he was . . . and then more
truth hit me. I was not nice; I was a judgemental cow hiding
behind a big smile.

This time I thought about all the judgements I'd made
about everyone around me since the moment I'd arrived.
I judged their colourful clothes and the far-out things they
said. I judged their nakedness, their tattoos and their ability
to spend hours engaged in hugs.

I judged it all because they seemed free in ways that I was
not – and I was jealous.

I thought of how I feared the judgement of others, but

I was the one judging. I judged others, but mostly I judged myself.

I needed to pee. The rain had started again and there were no toilets in the sauna area. I climbed over the fence into the woods behind. I was climbing a fence. Naked.

I walked with bare feet on soft earth and breathed in the drops of water and felt them hit my body. I found a tree and squatted behind it.

After I finished peeing, I kept walking in the woods. I found a pond with ducks and I stood in the rain, watching them.

I felt such peace. Watching these animals on the water, the rain dropping gently. It felt so simple now. I didn't need to fit in. I didn't have to be with people if I didn't want to. I didn't have to plaster on a smile when I didn't want to. I didn't have to be fancied.

This felt like a thrilling revelation, in the woods: I did not have to be anything other than what I was.

After the sauna, I got dressed and lay in the chill-out tent filled with rugs and people lounging around like a scantily clad sixth-form common room.

I found an unoccupied rug and sat on it, not quite sure what to do.

I didn't have my phone. Or a book. It was just me. Alone in a room full of people chatting to each other.

Feel this, I thought. Feel this discomfort. Don't run from it.

How many situations had I avoided out of fear of looking uncool, unpopular, like a loser? Again. Enough.

If I sat here alone like Billy No Mates for the rest of the day, who cared? I looked around at the tent of people lounging. There was another woman on her own, she was reading a book. It was called *Attached*, a book that Daisy had given me months ago and which I'd only flicked through. I could go and ask her about it, to make conversation, I thought. But why? I didn't want to make conversation just for the sake of not sitting on my own.

I was OK with how I was.

Alone.

And as soon as I thought that, a man sat down next to me.

Tall, pony-tailed . . . hot. I could see the outline of two nipple rings under his T-shirt.

He introduced himself. I introduced myself back.

'I saw you in the sauna, you looked serene,' he said.

'Did I?' I asked. 'Actually, I've been in a shit mood all day.'

He nodded like this was deeply fascinating and also normal.

'Would you like to get some food? I was going to get some dhal.'

And this is how it works in the hippy festival world apparently. You walk up to a stranger on a rug by a naked sauna and ask if they want a curry.

I said yes.

On the way to dinner we bumped into Daisy, who knew Jake, from her 'Buddhist days'. Anytime I was out with her, she knew somebody. In East London. Soho. A field in Suffolk. Daisy seemed to have lived a dozen lives. There were her Buddhist days, her clubbing days – and that time she thought she'd be an actress and got a bit part on an E4 show that got cancelled.

Surprisingly, I knew people too. I saw Hawaiian Santa sitting on a deckchair reading a Barbara Cartland book under a Crocodile Dundee hat.

'Is it good?' I asked him, pointing at the book.

'It does the job,' he smiled.

I introduced him to Daisy and Jake.

Before I knew it, I was in teenage heaven, finally feeling part of the cool gang.

For the next two days I existed in an idyll of touch and grass and sky and food and dancing. I lay on hammocks that hung between trees decorated with wind chimes. I danced in the woods. I played with children with painted faces. I met Jake's friends, who seemed like a big loose intergenerational family. They were wholesome in their openness, their intimacy looked natural and easy and unforced, and they all seemed to be connected.

Many lived in what they called a 'conscious community' – a big shared house in the Midlands where they shared meals and chores and childcare. I always thought of house-shares as being a studenty, twenty-something thing, but these people were forming an alternative family, with all ages from babies to sixty-somethings living together.

I wondered whether I'd be able to do that, or whether I'd miss having my own door to close.

I was introduced to a woman with a pregnancy bump and wild curly hair. She was at the festival with her husband and her girlfriend.

One of her friends was asking her about the wedding.

'It was great. We got married in a church but we asked the vicar not to mention God because Jez doesn't believe.'

'And the vicar agreed to that?' I asked. I couldn't believe it.

'Yes!' she smiled.

'And so you're married but you live with your girlfriend too?' I checked.

'Yes . . . Jez is my husband, and Ali is a lover and she lives with us. Which is great because Jez works long hours and I've had a lot of sickness during the pregnancy so it's great that Ali is there to bring me cups of tea or go shopping or whatever.'

My mind wanted to find fault with this arrangement. To find that actually it was dysfunctional – and yet this woman radiated joy. My mind was a ticker tape of questions.

'Have you always had more than one partner?' I asked.

'I was monogamous for many years, and I always ended up cheating and feeling terrible about it. When I met Jez I explained that I would always need more than one lover in my life and he said he was fine with that.'

'Wow.'

'We used to be with another couple but now it's just the three of us and that works well. I think my sexuality is happiest in a three but I usually like being with two men, so this is unusual. We're just making it up as we go along.'

She explained that to her polyamory wasn't a lifestyle choice, it was an innate part of her sexuality.

'It was too strong to ignore – and when I tried to ignore it, it caused me harm and pain and it caused other people harm and pain. And when I started to accept myself as I am, and allowed myself to do what I felt I needed to do, everything started to flow and I stopped causing people harm and pain. Suddenly my life was easy and lovely.'

'Are you as happy as you seem?' I asked.

She looked surprised by the question.

'I don't know how I seem – but yes, I'm happy,' she said.

'How do you get to be like this?'

'I was very loved as a child,' she replied.

I didn't think I'd ever heard anyone say that sentence before. What more could you ask for?

'Do your parents know?' I asked.

'Yeah, they don't understand,' she said. 'But that's OK.'

She smiled again.

———

When I left her I wandered around the festival on my own for a while, taking in the fact that there were so many ways to live life – many of them on show here.

I thought of terms I'd heard for the first time at the sologamy event. One of the women there had described herself as a 'relationship anarchist', which was new to me. It meant treating romantic and non-romantic relationships as if they had the same importance in your life. In other words, there isn't a hierarchy formed with your partner at the top and everyone else below.

'If me and my flatmate don't fancy each other but we both want a kid, why couldn't we be parents together?' asked one of the women at the event.

I'd heard a woman complaining about the 'relationship escalator', which was also new to me. I discovered it meant the track you traditionally got on when you met someone, moving up the commitment stakes from dating to sex to moving in to marriage to kids. Once you got on the escalator, it could be hard to get off. You just generally followed it to the top. It was a brilliant phrase that explained why I panicked as soon as I started dating anyone. It was like our whole potential future hung over the pub table, making it impossible for me to act normally.

Asexuality, on the other hand, I'd heard before but didn't know much about. It was a sexual orientation characterized by no or low level of interest in sexual activity with others. Asexual people may still form deep emotional connections and experience romantic attraction, and it wasn't the same as celibacy. At the time, I'd felt intimidated by these new ways of doing things, and my mind had not yet opened up to a world beyond the traditional. But it was beginning to.

I bumped into Jim the Builder, my tent neighbour, who

had just come from a drag workshop. 'I wore a dress and fishnets. My name was Beautiful Babs.'

There was still a trace of eyeliner under his eyes and sparkles on his cheeks. He looked beautiful and I told him so.

He introduced me to the woman he was with. They'd just got talking at the workshop. She was in her sixties and wasn't wearing the traditional hippy gear – she had cropped hair, three-quarter-length floral trousers and a blue T-shirt. She could have been on her way to Waitrose.

We sat down on the grass and talked. She was a retired teacher who had been diagnosed with cancer a couple of years before. When she was undergoing treatment she'd been told by friends to remember the good times and to know they would come again.

'I realized I'd never had any good times,' she said. 'And so I promised myself that if I got well that would change . . . so here I am! I got my boobs cut off, quit the job and left my husband.' She'd bought herself a campervan and was driving around the country visiting friends. In a few months her best friend was going to join her and they would drive around Europe together.

'I'd love to do that,' I said.

'What's stopping you?' she asked.

I didn't know. What *was* stopping me? Probably the idea that a real adult life meant staying at home and working and paying bills and not gallivanting around Europe? But if it was just me and I could work from anywhere – why didn't I do that?

'We might get married, actually,' she said. 'When my divorce is through. She has an Irish passport and I have an English one, and we were talking about retiring together in Spain or Italy and what with Brexit, it might be difficult for me.'

'Wow!'

'Well, we've known each other since we were six, so we know what we're getting into.'

'And do you fancy each other?'

She burst out laughing.

'God, no! But never say never!'

'Would you like a tantric massage?' Jake asked on the final afternoon.

We'd been hanging out for two days and I fancied him, but was pretending not to. I assumed he didn't fancy me and was just one of those chat-to-everyone types. Even when he asked me if I'd like a massage I didn't know if this was just something you did if you lived in a conscious community house share. A bit like asking someone if they wanted a cup of tea.

It was such a clean, straightforward offer. I said yes and we went back to his tent and he laid down a huge sarong over his blow-up mattress.

I felt nervous. Should I get undressed? Or not? It was 2 p.m. and I was potentially getting naked with a man with two nipple rings in a tent. This was not normal. But no, Marianne, come on . . . this is the point, to get past normal.

I took off all my clothes except my knickers.

He unpacked squeezy bottles of coconut oil from his backpack and said, 'There's nothing you need to do, just relax.'

And I did. Relax. More than I usually did with a hot man.

Usually when I'm with someone I fancy, I'm locked in my head thinking of what I should be doing and worrying if it was good enough. I'm too busy worrying about my performance to enjoy anything. Being told that there was nothing I needed to do was a gift – just as it had been at tantra.

And so I spent the morning being touched in ways I had

never been touched before. I asked him to take off my knickers.

At one point his slippery hands turned into a slippery chest and his whole body was moving up mine in a greasy heaven and noises were coming out of me that I did not know could come out of me. Deep, animal sounds. For a second I worried about people hearing through the tent. Then I didn't care.

'How did you learn to do that?' I asked afterwards.

He had done a lot of 'work' around sexuality, including tantric massage courses.

He was an advert for it.

I swear if everyone in the world knew how to touch like he did, there would be no wars. We'd all be too busy moaning in tents and gazing at butterflies and oozing like honey.

I wanted more.

On the last night we all – Daisy, Jim the Builder, Jake and his friends, Hawaiian Santa and my other tantra friends – went to the dance tent.

The music was a pounding bass and the tent was full of people dancing together and alone, eyes closed or wide open.

At first, I felt stiff and awkward compared to these uninhibited creatures but soon my body moved on its own, responding to the beat, moving in sync with everyone around me. It was bliss. To be a human in a body that danced. To be part of the crowd.

This was why people came to festivals. This transcendent togetherness. To be one.

My body hummed and my heart pounded. I was alive. Everything felt right. I was a human body moving with other human bodies.

I danced with Jim, who was no longer a builder but a raving sprite.

'Say what you like about hippies,' he shouted in my ear, 'but they throw a good party!'

These weird hippies weren't weird at all. This was how we should be living – outdoors, together, with singing and dancing and trees and good food and fires and mysticism and grass, and it was so simple, it took so little – why have we gone so far from this life? And why did this life feel like a delusion and a fairy tale, and normal life feel real? It was normal life that was so unreal – a life of screens and seeking validation from people you'd never met, of putting on your best show on Instagram by day and watching serial killers by night.

By the time we drove home I was quite sure I'd found paradise. I wanted to live in this Garden of Eden with smiling, shining, serene people with willy rings and fairy wings. This was it! A life of freedom and joy and slippery coconut-oil bodies! A life with no inhibitions and singing and dancing and vegetable dhal! This was the life I wanted! I wanted to fuck in the woods! Lie in mud! Sing by fires inhaling the smell of burning wood under the night sky! This was life. Yes, this.

In the car, I made resolutions. I was going to look after myself more, remember that my body was a sacred vessel and let pure divine light shine through every pore.

Maybe I'd get a campervan and drive around Europe. And become a vegan. Maybe I'd move into Jake's conscious community, and live a life of vegetable chopping rotas and sexual ecstasy.

8

Summer of Love

'His name is Jake and he's training to be a sexological body-worker,' I said.

'What's that?'

'It's someone who works with people's bodies in a way that includes their sexuality.' I repeated the phrase that he had given me.

'You mean he's a sex worker?'

'No, he's actually a plumber. But he's doing this stuff on the side.'

'So is he going to be your wax on, wax off sex guru?' Rachel asked.

'Maybe.'

'Did you like him?'

'Yeah. I really did. He's the most honest person I've ever met – he told me my breath was bad and that he could smell my armpits.'

'What?'

I laughed. 'I know, it's full-on, but it was refreshing. He showed me what deodorant he uses, he actually took it out of his bag to show me.'

'What was it?'

'Some natural one that smelled of cloves.'

'I tried those rock ones for a while, they were useless.'

'Yeah. Me too. And he told me he never wanted to be in a monogamous relationship.'

Rachel rolled her eyes.

'I know, I know but honestly this festival was so beautiful, it was like a whole other world. Everyone looked so happy. I met a woman who was there with her husband *and* her girlfriend. The three of them were just hanging out together. They all seemed so –' I tried to find the word that summed it up, 'free. Yes. Free. That's it.'

And I wanted to be free. I wanted to be free from body hang-ups, free from sexual hang-ups, free from hang-ups about what people thought of me . . .

We were at Hampstead Heath by the ladies' pond. Teenage girls were lying on laid-out towels in various states of undress with a portable speaker playing tinny music I didn't know.

'Would you like to be that young again?' I asked Rachel.

'Sometimes. Things were easier then, you just had fun and didn't think about anything.'

'I was too scared to have fun when I was their age.'

'You're having your teenage rebellion aged forty,' said Rachel.

I laughed. That was exactly what I was doing.

Rachel wasn't in her teenage rebellion – she had had her second egg retrieval and it had been disappointing.

'I'm sorry,' I said.

She shrugged. 'What you gonna do?' she asked. It was the thing she always said when stuff was going wrong.

'Get drunk and forget?' Which was what I always said when things were going wrong.

'I can't drink with the hormones.'

'Oh yeah.'

I didn't know what to say to make her feel better. Maybe

there was nothing to say. I told her how brilliant I thought she was for doing this. She said thanks.

'Shall we go for a swim?' I asked, after a few minutes of silence.

'I don't think I will, you go.'

'Are you sure? I'm happy to just hang out here.'

'No, it's OK, go and I'll look after our things.'

There were queues to get in the water. It was a hot summer and every flat-dweller in the city had found their way to a park.

I looked at all the female bodies on show. The flat tummies of teenage girls, the lean bodies of young yoga mothers, the heft and jiggle of older women who had seen it all before and glided through the water like queens. A woman with long, white hair pinned into a bun was being helped into the water from a wheelchair. All of womanhood was here, and we were magnificent in our relaxation.

For the first time ever, I did not compare my body to those around me.

The water was cold silk, and for a while I swam without any thoughts. When I reached a buoy in the middle of the pond I lay on my back and looked at the sky. This was it, I thought. This was what life was about. This. Being a body in the water and a sky up above. Feeling the sun on my limbs. Enjoying life. Enjoying the summer. How many summers I'd missed in offices or fretting over deadlines. This would be my summer . . . of love. The teenage summer I never had. A summer of no responsibilities.

I thought about Jake and smiled. I couldn't remember where he said he'd be right now. A field somewhere. I tried not to think about whether he'd be giving massages to other women. Although, so what if he was?

Then I thought about Rachel and how much she was

handling on her own. I was not being a good friend by constantly running off on retreats and festivals.

I swam back to her. She was frowning at her phone.

'Are you OK?' I asked.

'I've been getting a rash where I'm injecting the hormones and I've been googling to see if it's normal, and I end up on chat rooms full of women talking about their "darling husbands" or "lovely boyfs" doing the injections for them.'

I stuck out my tongue at the terms. 'So *is* it normal?' I asked.

'I don't know, I stopped reading – I already feel like a freak for having to do this and all the stuff online is geared towards couples. I went for a scan the other day and the receptionist saw me sitting in one chair and my rucksack was on the chair next to me, and she asked me, "Where has he gone?"'

'Oh god.'

'Yeah. I mean I laughed, it was funny but – like, what should I say? "Actually, he went off with a woman called Emma and had a lovely baby naturally! Even though he told me he didn't want children!" Sorry. I'm shit company.'

'You're not, it's OK.'

'I'm spending my days sticking needles in my stomach at the kitchen table wondering how the fuck this is my life. Last weekend I went to a wedding and I had to inject hormones when I was there so I packed them in a picnic bag with frozen peas to keep them cold. I sat there on the loo injecting myself praying I wouldn't fuck it up and get blood on my dress.'

I laughed. 'Sorry, it's not funny.'

'No, it is,' she said. 'Kind of. Anyway, enough of that. What are you reading?'

'Don't change the subject,' I said.

'I want to, please, let me think of something else,' she said.

I held up my book. *The Ethical Slut.*

'Jake recommended it. It's meant to be a free-love bible.'

'Why do they have to use that word?'

'They're reclaiming it, like how the *Pussy* woman is reclaiming "pussy". I quite like it.'

'I don't,' she said, picking at the grass. 'So do you think you could do it?'

'What?'

'See different people at the same time.'

'Yes, it makes sense to me . . . we have different friends in our lives and it's not a problem. It actually makes more sense to me than dating and looking for one person that has to be your everything, and that's hanging in the room every time you meet some random guy off an app – how can you be normal in that scenario? At least I can't. I dunno. There's so much pressure on it . . . It's like on the tantra workshops you can hug and kiss and touch people without it having to mean anything – I really like it, it takes off all the heaviness . . . things can just be in the moment, there's no weight on it, and actually then beautiful things happen with the most unexpected people.'

Rachel looked at me like I was speaking Russian.

'I knew someone who was in a poly relationship. He said they spent all their time having conversations about their feelings – and updating Google calendars.'

'Yeah. I don't know what I'd do with all that side of things.'

'I am not going to manage your diary if you get into this,' she said. I laughed.

'So are you going to see the festival guy again?' she asked.

'Yeah, I hope so, but he's away most of the summer. He asked me how much I want to be in touch.'

'Did you tell him you never answer your phone?' she asked.

'No, but I told him that I wasn't a big communicator. He

said he liked to be in contact but that I shouldn't feel any pressure to reply to all the messages he sends.'

Rachel took this in. 'Wow.'

'I know.'

'It's just so . . . respectful.'

'Yeah.'

'And simple.'

'Yeah.'

'Just to ask like that. How much do you want to be in touch . . .'

'I know! He's done a lot of therapy. Everything is kind of just said out loud.'

We were both silent at the idea of that.

'OK, I need to prepare for a pitch, and then I've got a date,' Rachel said, getting up from her towel.

'Tonight?'

'Yes.'

'Are you sure you're up to it?'

'I can't let my life stop,' she snapped.

I wanted to tell her to rest, and that maybe she was not in the best headspace to make small talk with a stranger, but I didn't.

'You're getting into polyamory and I'd settle for just amory,' she said as she kissed me goodbye.

I once saw a guy reading a copy of the Kama Sutra in a pub in Soho. Wanker, I thought. Does that really work?

Well, yes it does.

For the rest of the summer, I sat in various London parks waiting for my sexual liberation to come. I didn't have to wait long – turns out it helps to be holding a book with the word 'slut' in the title.

The Ethical Slut: A Practical Guide to Polyamory, Open Relationships and Other Adventures in Sex and Love is a bible for polyamory. Written by Janet W. Hardy and Dossie Easton – who describe themselves as friends, colleagues and lovers – it outlines a free-love utopia.

From the second page I wanted to be their best friend, buy a plane ticket and move in with them in San Francisco. The world they described seemed so . . . wholesome. It was an unexpected word to use for a book that tells you what to wear at a sex party, but that was the vibe: wholesome, shame-free joy.

Hardy and Easton define a 'slut' as 'a person of any gender who has the courage to lead life according to the radical proposition that sex is nice and pleasure is good for you'. They advocate for a different model of relationships: a world where we love and respect each other just as we are – without trying to fit people into boxes marked 'partner'.

'Are you polyamorous?' a slight, dark-haired man asked from the next table in a coffee shop.

'No,' I said, embarrassed at how far from polyamorous I was. 'I'm hardly amorous,' I replied, stealing Rachel's line.

He smiled. He was visiting London from San Francisco where the 'poly scene' was popular with his tech friends.

I looked at him. He was shorter than me. Skinny. I thought that if I sat on his lap I would crush him. Within seconds I had come up with at least a dozen reasons why this man was not relationship material, including the fact that he wore those trainers that looked like gloves, the ones where all his toes showed.

Every encounter with a man led to this flash-second analysis of whether this guy would be The One – was this someone I wanted to spend the rest of my life with? Was he hot enough, clever enough? Tall enough? Funny enough?

Would my friends like him? If he was any of those things, I was so intimidated I ran a mile. And the fact that I was deeply ambivalent about the idea of The One didn't even seem to matter. I still put men through this checklist. It was so weighted that any flame was snuffed instantly.

Regular, non-slutty me would have smiled at him in a way that made it very clear I didn't want to talk more, and would get back to my book. But what did I miss out on by doing this? And how brutal was it to hold people up to these arbitrary standards and then toss them aside? There were a million standards I didn't live up to.

The Ethical Slut told me to see the beauty in everyone. Tantra had shown me that this was possible. On my first retreat I'd had beautiful connections with the most unexpected people: Hawaiian Santa, er-Jay the Ipswich hugger. People who were older and younger and not my 'type'.

'My name's Marianne,' I said.

He told me his name. He said he had been spending his time visiting the best coffee shops in London.

I wondered why we were all so obsessed with coffee these days.

He said he didn't know.

He told me he'd been to a show and was going to a concert tonight.

'Who are you seeing?'

'New Order. They're playing somewhere called Alexandra Palace tonight, do you want to come?' he asked.

I looked at my phone. It was 4 p.m. already.

'Tonight?'

'Yeah.'

'I doubt there are tickets left,' I said.

He went onto StubHub.

Four hours later we were shouting along: 'Love will tear us apart again . . .'

I sang my heart out and he did too. We got talking to a couple dancing next to us. They'd met at a New Order gig when they were students, and now paid for a babysitter every time New Order played. They looked so young bouncing up and down. I thought about the power of music to make us feel like the best version of ourselves, and realized that I had danced more in these last few months than I had in my whole life. I loved it.

Dancing in the crowd, I had the same feeling of possibility I had when I was travelling. When I was abroad I said yes to things without overthinking them. I could go out with men without the whole '*What is this?*' thing hanging in the air. It didn't matter. I was just a human liking another human at that moment. And far from being empty and false, actually these connections felt true and deep.

On the bus home he asked if I wanted to come back to his Airbnb. I said I didn't and he seemed fine with it. When he got off at his stop, he kissed me on the cheek and thanked me for a great evening.

It was so straightforward. If he was disappointed by my 'no' he didn't show it. In fact I wondered if he might have been relieved. We'd had a lovely night and it didn't need anything more.

'So your first night as a slut and you go home on your own?' Rachel replied, when I texted her to tell her I was home safe.

'Yes!' I said. With no disappointment.

In fact, the book says that you can be a celibate slut or an asexual slut. Sluttery is about what goes on in your head more than what goes on between your legs.

And I was becoming a slut in my head.

———

Something happened that summer. It seemed that every man
I'd ever had an encounter with came out of the woodwork.
Guys I knew as a teenager would message to say, 'Hey . . .
long time . . .' People I met when travelling got in touch to say
they might be in town. Male friends who'd broken up with
their girlfriends started texting to ask to go for a drink. It was
like I was sending out some siren call.

First to get in contact was a man I'd met travelling the
States a few years earlier. He messaged every now and then
and his tone was always flirty. I generally replied with questions about how his job was going.

'What are you wearing?' he asked on Facebook Messenger.

'Not much,' I replied, which was actually true. The flat was
like a greenhouse and I was sitting by my laptop in my underwear by a fan, with a wet towel over my shoulders.

He sent me a picture of his erection inside his shorts.

I imagined there was a sexy emoji I should use in times like
this but I hadn't got the memo.

'Oh!' I replied.

'Send me a pic?' he asked.

'No,' I replied.

'Do you want to video?' he asked.

My instinct reaction was no. No, I do not! How very dare
you! I am a reputable woman who cannot just be ordered like
a takeaway! I was worth more than that!

But was I? What did that even mean: to be worth more
than that? *The Ethical Slut* talked about how messed up it was
that sex was traded like a commodity and that it was women's
job to hold back in order to make themselves more valuable.
I thought about how much a woman's sexuality was wrapped
up in the language of commerce – cheap, worthless, trash. It
was bullshit.

The truth was, I felt excited and wanted to see this man

again. I wanted to have phone sex . . . or Skype sex . . . or Facebook sex . . . whatever medium we were going to use. It was something I'd never done before.

'Yes,' I replied before I could find reasons not to. I quickly tidied up my bed, changed into my Greek underwear and took my hair down.

The video call came through on Facebook.

I pressed to answer but it kept ringing.

'It won't let me answer,' I messaged in the chat box.

'What browser are you using?' he typed.

'Safari.'

'Download Chrome or Firefox.'

'OK, give me ten.'

I downloaded Chrome, and then I couldn't log in to Facebook because I couldn't remember my password, which was saved on Safari. I went back to my Safari browser.

'I can't get on FB on Chrome.'

'Let's do Skype.'

The Skype ringtone started and this time I could answer. He appeared on the screen, this man I'd met in a hotel years before.

'Hi,' I said. 'It's nice to see you.'

'I can't hear you,' he said.

'Oh, that's weird.'

'I can't hear you. Is your volume off?'

'No, it's up high,' I said, speaking louder.

He started texting me instructions for how to check the microphone settings.

I did what he suggested and it didn't work.

'Try switching your computer off and back on again.'

I was in my Greek underwear on a call with the IT help desk.

Five minutes later we were back on the screen with the volume working.

It was clear he had done this before; he knew the best angle to make him look big. He reached out to pretend he was touching my boobs. It was unexpectedly hot and I surprised myself by getting into my first on-screen performance.

It was only afterwards, when I shut my laptop, that fear hit. What if he had been recording? What if he sent it out around the world? But what if he did? I hadn't done anything wrong. I was a single woman having phone sex with a single man. So what? What was there to be ashamed of?

But I was ashamed.

I felt that he had somehow got the upper hand. But why was that the case? He had asked me to join him, and I had. Because I'd wanted to. And that was the bit I found uncomfortable. I'd wanted it.

The Ethical Slut says, 'To be truly free to explore our sexual potential to the fullest, most of us need to examine how we have been taught that someone of our gender is supposed to enjoy sex.'

The answer was easy – women were not meant to just want and enjoy sex. They were supposed to want the committed relationship and sex was only a way of getting there, or would only be enjoyable, meaningful or 'good' if it was with a man who loved you and was committed to you.

And what if you weren't angling for the long-term relationship? Did that mean you were supposed to be sexless? That was how I'd been living my life.

Hardy and Easton say, 'We see ourselves surrounded by the walking wounded – by people who have been injured by fear, shame and hatred of their own sexual selves.' The solution was simple: 'We believe that happy, guilt-free connection is the cure for their wounds; we believe that sex and intimacy

are vital to people's sense of self-worth. To their belief that
life is good.'

And so I spent the rest of the summer trying to live by this
idea: sex was good, and so was life.

The next week, Daisy and I went to a deliciously air-
conditioned art gallery and sat at the bar. Her post break-up
stint on my blow-up bed was over – she had moved into
a room in a friend's house-share in Hackney Wick and I
missed her.

'The barman keeps looking at you,' Daisy said as we
got a drink before pretending to be cultured. I looked over
at him.

'Don't be stupid, he's a child.'

'He's into you,' she insisted.

After the show we went back to the bar where the
barman gave us two free drinks and told us about a party
happening down the road. Did we want to go with him?
We did.

I felt eighty years older than the shiny-faced twenty-
somethings around me. The barman didn't tell me his age
but he had only recently graduated from university. I was old
enough to be his mother, literally.

Did that matter?

The Ethical Slut would argue not. 'We believe that all relationships have the potential to teach us, move us, and above
all give us pleasure. We believe it's OK to have sex with
anybody you love, and we believe in loving everybody,' the
authors say.

He lived a couple of roads away from me. We got an Uber
home together. I was drunk. Too drunk to feel or remember

very much of our night together, beyond him being gentle and asking for consent in a way no man my age had ever done.

The next morning he asked if I wanted his number.

'No pressure,' he said. 'But it would be nice to hang out again.'

He was more mature than I was, but I didn't know whether to take this any further.

Hardy and Easton argue that in today's world we act like there is nothing between 'emotionless sport fucking and committed long-term marriage-type relationships' – but actually there is 'a vast territory in between open to discovery'.

The book says that relationships seek their own level and we should just let them be whatever they are meant to be. Some connections will last a lifetime, some just a few minutes. Some will turn into friendships, some into passionate affairs. All could be worthwhile and have great value. I loved this way of thinking.

I put his number into my phone.

The book argues that polyamory can be a great way to work through feelings of sexual inadequacy because through experience with different kinds of people you learn a lot and you see that 'great lovers are made, not born. You can learn from your lovers, and your lovers' lovers, and your lovers' lovers' lovers, to become the sexual superstars you want to be!'

We saw each other a few more times. He was lovely, and I wanted to learn. But I was coming up against a few blocks:

To be sexual I had to be drunk, and this, I realized, meant I felt very little physically.

When he asked what I liked, I honestly didn't know, which

meant that we seemed to get stuck in this formulaic paint-by-numbers approach to sex: snog, fiddle, penetration.

Anytime I was in bed, my mind was narrating the whole thing, telling me that I was doing everything wrong.

I was shy of the male body – in particular the penis.

Penetration often felt uncomfortable. Not painful exactly, though it could be, but not enjoyable. I put on noises pretending I enjoyed it and waited for it to be over.

I was getting notches on the bedpost, which was good for my ego, but I was nowhere near the transcendent sex I craved – or even the melty, honey feeling I'd experienced with Jake in the tent, or on my first tantra retreat.

Sometimes it felt like we were two can openers in bed together.

And the reason it felt awkward was obvious: I was bad at sex.

I went back to my therapist.

'I didn't know what a Virgin Mary I was around sex,' I said.

'Didn't you?' she replied. (Are therapists allowed to be sarcastic?) 'And who would you be if you weren't a Virgin Mary?' she asked.

'I dunno . . .' I looked out of the window behind her and thought about it . . . 'I'd be free – I'd be able to have great sex, and to have fights when I'm pissed off and travel the world and not give a fuck.'

'That sounds fun,' she said. For our next session she asked me to come as my alter ego, the part of myself that I repress.

I arrived at her Hampstead house in a mac and high heels. My Greek underwear underneath.

I felt powerful. Grown-up.

As soon as the session was over, I changed back into my normal jeans and baggy top.

I had to face this. I wanted to get over my shame. And get good at sex.

9

Sex School

'Did you bring lube?' Hawaiian Santa asked a tall man wearing a fleece.

'I brought coconut oil. What about you?'

'Same.'

They looked at me.

'Er, no, I forgot,' I said.

'I'm sure they'll have some there,' the tall guy said.

'Yeah,' I said, tummy flipping at the horror of what was ahead.

A mess of hot chocolate, wooden sticks, emptied sugar sachets and coffee cups sat between us. Kids were screaming on the brown pleather sofa next to our table. Their grandparents looked like they'd been run over. The sprawling Costa we were sitting in, in Staines felt like suburban Armageddon. And the most unlikely place to be making small talk about lube, about to head off and have sex with strangers – and maybe each other.

I had signed up to another tantra retreat. This one seemed to be more explicitly sexual. And you had to have done the first one to join this second, more advanced one.

It was taking place in Somerset and emails had been sent around with people offering lifts, which was why three of us were meeting in the Costa in Staines.

The email sent out had encouraged us to bring 'your own

intimate lubricant and/or a jar of coconut oil. There may be times when you would find that useful.'

The idea petrified me so much that I'd closed my laptop and wiped it from my memory.

'Actually, I might run to Superdrug now and get some,' I said.

I made my way out of the cafe and went to Superdrug, past teenagers hanging outside Staines shopping centre. I bought Mitchum max strength deodorant and witch hazel for the spot that was developing on my cheek. I didn't have the courage to ask the woman in a headscarf behind the till where the lube was. I ran back to the cafe, where our lift was waiting. We packed our sarong- and towel-filled bags and made our way onto the M25. Four almost strangers listening to Heart FM in a Fiat Uno, on their way to sex school.

Once there, we signed another condom contract and I told them, again, that I didn't like mushrooms. The week started, again, with sober dancing, this time under the watchful gaze of a papier-mâché dragon who was popping out of the wall of the hall, like a badly made film prop.

The condom hors d'oeuvres were there again, twinkling in their Quality Street wrappers. Jan was there again too, in her head-to-toe colours and Madonna mic. Once we sat down in the opening circle we were told where we could smoke, where the recycling was and what to do if the fire alarm went off.

Last point of housekeeping: we were not to hug the chef. 'He doesn't like it,' said Jan, before telling us what this week was about.

There were fifty of us in the room – some familiar faces, many new ones. 'The invitation is to treat this like school,' said Jan. 'This is a chance to learn the things you were never taught. There is no such thing as 'I should know this by now' – this is where we come to learn together. Be curious – and never push yourself too far.'

The idea was that we were not born knowing how to do sex. It was a skill that we cultivated through practice and learning. Great lovers were not born, they were made, as the *Ethical Slut* authors put it.

And so began seven days in the Big Brother tantra house. Seven days that were the sex education I never got. Seven days I didn't think, at several points, I'd get through.

At first it was OK. More sober dancing. More sitting in circles and having excruciating conversations. There was an exercise where we were invited to act out different kinds of sex, from duty sex to holy sex, in a kind of x-rated am-dram. I got through it all with only mild chest pains and then . . . well, then the real stuff started. Jan offered us the opportunity to practise something or try something that we'd always wanted to try. She explained that it might be that we wanted to practise putting a condom on someone. Or . . . well, I didn't hear what she said next, I was too busy trying not to vomit.

I knew what I needed to practise. I knew what I had a real block around. I knew that this was the place to face my fear of . . .

No, I couldn't. No, no, no.

I ran out to the toilet. I tried to breathe. I looked at myself in the mirror.

'Pull yourself together, fucking pull yourself together.'

My face was sweaty and red, and a spot on my cheek was throbbing.

I walked out of the toilet to find Hawaiian Santa waiting in line.

I burst into tears. Santa ducked into one of the toilets and passed me some toilet roll.

'Thank you.'

'Are you all right?'

'No.'

'Would you like a cup of tea?'

'No. Yes. OK. Yes.'

'Why don't I make tea and you sit outside and get some air?'

'OK.'

I walked out to a bench by the kitchen wall, overlooking a courtyard and a garden. I kept my head down.

Santa (whose real name was Matthew) came back, sat next to me and passed me a tea.

'Thank you.'

'You're welcome.'

'I hate this,' I said.

'Hate what?' he asked.

'How bad I am at all this.'

'All what?'

'This. Sex stuff.'

He nodded and kept looking at me, like a hippy priest.

'When everyone was in their teens and twenties learning how to do things, I was just too scared. All I ever had were messy drunken encounters. I feel like I missed that whole bit where you just learn. I always have this feeling – that I'm not good enough. That I'm doing it wrong, that I'm letting men down.'

'You can't do anything wrong. Just be present, that's all anyone wants.'

'But I don't know what to do,' I said, and felt my eyes

welling up. 'I don't know what to do with . . .' Oh my god, was I going to say this?

His eyes kept looking at me.

'I don't know what to do with a penis.'

And there it was. My shameful secret.

Ever since attempting my first hand-job at university, when the guy asked me to please stop, I froze when it came to touching these alien appendages. I felt relaxed with oral sex, funnily enough, but when it came to touching the penis I felt panicked and frozen . . . so much that I often skipped to penetrative sex much sooner than I wanted so that I could skip the fiddling-around bit.

It felt so shameful to say that, so raw and so young. How had I let it come to this? To feel so inadequate at this age. It was humiliating.

'But that's why we're here, to learn,' he said, taking my hand.

'I have this idea that everyone else is really good at it – that like, you're all cool with everything and you're like these sex gurus and I'm like this stupid child. But I'm forty!'

'I don't think anyone is here because they think they're a sex guru,' smiled Santa.

'I'd like to practise touching a penis.' I could not believe I had uttered those words. 'Could you help me?'

'It would be my honour.'

'Are you sure?'

'Yes.'

'Thank you.' Then: 'Are you just saying that to be nice and because you feel you have to?'

'No,' he said.

I started crying. 'I'm sorry,' I said.

'Don't be. Your tears are the river we swim to meet you,' he said.

We sat in silence as I cried and he held my hand and the sun shone on our faces.

'Would you mind?' he asked, moving his finger towards my cheek. I nodded. He wiped my tears away.

'That was a very good line – about the tears and river,' I said.

'I try,' he smiled.

We walked back in.

When the moment came, Matthew took off his trousers, boxers and specs.

'I'm too sexy for my glasses,' he smiled, and I laughed.

I didn't feel the panic I'd expected. I had seen his body before and I felt safe with it, with him.

One of the female teachers said she would join us and show me various techniques. Watching her touch him was like watching poetry in motion, she danced her fingers around his cock. It was spellbinding. There wasn't a bicycle pump motion in sight.

She showed me different moves: the pulling the endless handkerchief out of a hat move, where you pull from the base of the penis up the shaft and off with one hand and then the other, and on and on. Juicing a lemon: where you massage the top of the penis – as the name suggests – as though you're juicing a lemon. Pushing the penis round and round, like a helicopter – I couldn't believe that that didn't hurt, but apparently it doesn't when the penis is not erect.

Then it was my turn. I started with the helicopter, then moved on to stroking and juicing the lemon . . .

My sexy talk started. *You don't know what you're doing, you fucking idiot, you are forty and you still don't know what you're doing, what a loser, you're doing it wrong, your hands are sweaty and clammy and shaking and everyone else finds this easy, you freak, no man in their right mind would ever fancy you . . .*

And then I looked up and saw that Matthew was smiling.

He's just smiling to be nice. He pities you. He doesn't understand how you can be so bad at this.

But then I looked up at Matthew again, who was beaming now. *Oh – maybe this is going OK! I can do this!*

From then on, I let go of the chatter. I touched him how I wanted to touch him, I didn't think about getting it right or wrong, I just breathed and breathed and let my hands dance on his skin . . . I just moved my fingers where they wanted to go . . . then I even started to have fun! He opened his eyes and gave me two thumbs-up like a children's TV presenter and it was funny and a relief, and afterwards he said, 'That was really good.'

'You're just saying that,' I said.

'I'm not – honestly. I am not.'

I was delighted with myself.

And then we swapped and he gave me a yoni massage – a spiritual version of Rachel's idea of fingering – which gave me the giggles. It wasn't that anything was funny – although being at sex camp had the makings of a black comedy – it was more that my body was giggling involuntarily, like a spasm.

It felt innocent and sweet . . . and delightful.

Yes, that was it, it was delightful. Not sexy exactly, not erotic or edgy. Just delightful.

Matthew told me that I'd had a 'gigglegasm'.

'A what?'

He smiled. 'It's a thing!'

Bliss will come from the places you least want to go. I can't remember if someone told me that or if I'd seen it on Facebook, but it popped into my head.

I wondered how many situations I'd run away from for fear of showing weakness or of saying, 'I don't know what to do, can you show me?' to save face. How much my behaviour

had been driven by the fearful voice saying *I can't do that –
they'll think I'm an idiot or a loser.* The perpetual teenager
in my head. I thought about his assurance that all anyone
wanted was for the other person to be present.

High on my spiritual hand-job triumph, I dared to imagine
that maybe I could overcome my insecurities and become a
sexually liberated woman of the world! A master lover!

Dinner was mushroom stroganoff.

After that we were invited to share our sexual fantasies in
front of the whole group. I ran out of the room. It was too
much.

Jan had said that this was like school – and it was. I felt
like I was in an exam that I was failing. A teenage nightmare
I couldn't escape. It felt like this week encapsulated so much
of what I'd spent my life running from.

That night I sat in the dorm chatting with other women. At
first, the scenario made me feel stressed, just as it had at the
women's circle. Again, I remembered teenage sleepovers
where conversations would turn to boys and I would sit in
hot, prickly silence, wishing the floor would swallow me.

We talked about the messages we'd got about sex growing
up. Most of us had been told versions of 'boys only want one
thing', and 'girls who have sex are sluts, or "easy" '. It was our
job to say 'no'.

'When I went to my first dance my mother told me that
boys would "want to do things" and I was to say no and that
I'd be dirty if I didn't,' said an Irish woman in her late fifties.
'So when I was asked to dance I told all the boys to go away!
I kept telling them to go away – which is why I'm here now.'
She was funny, but it was not.

My roommate talked about 'doing too much too soon' to

get the attention of boys at school. 'I thought I was enjoy-ing it, but I wasn't. Not really. I was desperate for attention,' she said.

Another woman, in her early thirties, spoke with her head down. She described her first experience as being 'quite close to rape'.

The room was quiet as we gave her the opportunity to say something more. She didn't.

We talked about how sex education at school had never mentioned that sex could be nice and pleasurable and part of a loving relationship. Instead it was fear-based: do not get pregnant or contract an STI.

'I remember being told that if I got raped I had to keep the baby because that's what God would want,' I found myself saying.

I hadn't thought of that lesson since it had happened, but as I spoke, it came back clearly. I was sitting in RE at a desk by the window in the New Block while the teacher told us why abortion was wrong under any circumstances.

'But what if we get pregnant because we were raped?' some brave classmate asked.

'Then God wants you to have that baby,' the teacher explained.

It was only as I said it now, as an adult, that I realized how full on that was.

'Then all the AIDS awareness stuff started on television.' I remembered adverts with tombstones – the message was loud and clear: sex kills. It became clear in that moment that sex and rape and AIDS and pregnancy had all blended into one in my young teenage mind.

And so I had largely avoided men and sex. There were drunken encounters in my late teens and twenties, which were rarely enjoyable but served the purpose of allowing me to feel like I wasn't a complete weirdo. My lack of experience haunted me.

In my thirties I'd had relationships and I liked sex, but I still had the feeling of being inadequate. I thought that sex was another thing I should be 'good' at. It didn't really occur to me that sex could be something for my own enjoyment, not just something I did for someone else. It also never occurred to me that it was ridiculous to be expected to be good at something nobody had ever taught you how to do.

'We have all these recipes and books telling us how to make a roast chicken, whole Sunday supplements devoted to food, but nobody tells us how to touch someone,' I found myself saying. Suddenly it seemed ridiculous that we were so secretive and shameful about this really important part of life.

'I was listening to a podcast,' said the Irish woman. 'It was about sex education in Holland. They start at the age of four. Four! But it's not about what goes where, it's about relationships and friendships and how the kids might feel fuzzy around special friends. The sex gets introduced later but in the context of being with someone you really like. Apparently they have the highest rate of satisfaction for people's first time and the lowest teenage pregnancy rates.'

Most women in the room had not had a positive first experience.

That night I lay awake again, my mind a spin cycle of teenage memories I had not thought of in years. I thought of *More* magazine's Position of the Fortnight, read in my sixth-form common room, featuring cartoons of couples doing naked gymnastics. I didn't know if the girls who had boyfriends were having sex up against a washing machine, but by this point I hadn't even had my first proper kiss.

I'd felt like a loser.

I'd gone to an all-girls school, so boys were this other thing, this scary thing – I didn't have brothers. We met boys in town, in the shopping-centre years, and I was always too scared to get involved. And that had been the main feeling around boys and sex – fear.

Bad things will happen because of it. You'll get raped, you'll get pregnant, you'll get a disease – or people will laugh at you.

Because that was another thing I was always aware of – the jeering laughter of men, shouting on the street, 'Oh, wouldn't mind a bit of that.'

We were all considered to be a 'bit of stuff'.

Being pressured into sex didn't feel like a big deal back then – it was the norm. Kissing turned into groping and fumbling, which turned into sex because we didn't know how to stop it. We were warned not to be a 'prick-tease'. If you turned a boy on it was your responsibility to 'finish him off'.

And so, while my friends got their first boyfriends, I hid in my room listening to Tori Amos, nursing crushes from a safe distance. I liked unrequited love, it felt comfortable and satisfying and it was a good hurt, the kind you got from twisting baby teeth almost ready to drop out. Now, at forty, I still felt like that teenager hiding in her bedroom listening to Tori Amos.

And it wasn't just me. The next day in the big group room, people shared harrowing tales of rejection, shame, lack of confidence, and trauma. There was childhood abuse; toxic relationships; Victorian parenting; crippling shyness; physical embarrassment . . . I'd always thought that everyone else was cool when it came to sex. That they were at ease and 'normal' in ways that I was not. That turned out not to be the case. We were all carrying baggage. We were invited to use this week as an opportunity to talk about a subject that is usually shrouded in silence.

These were conversations I'd never had before. Not with my friends, not with anyone. It felt awkward and important to be having them. But it was hard too. I felt like I was facing up to things I'd spent a lifetime running away from.

By the second-to-last day I was feeling overwhelmed, so when we were told we were about to enter another 'structure' and that we should partner up, I asked the woman sitting next to me if she would like to work together.

'I need a break from men,' I said.

She said, 'Me too.'

Jan talked on her Madonna mic about how important it was to get in touch with our desires and to voice them, regardless of whether they ever happen or not. It's important to own our desires. It's also important as someone's partner to listen to those desires without shaming them, but also without feeling any pressure to oblige. This would be another chance to practise our yeses and nos.

I didn't know what my desires were.

As a woman, I thought my job was to be attractive enough to be the object of desire, and to be on guard for when that desire came from the wrong people, but my own desires . . . never came into it. I didn't know what my desires were. Even the word 'desire' – urgh – like moist and lover, it made me cringe. Desires felt wanting, greedy, unfeminine . . . dangerous. But then I remembered the fun of admitting my desires during Pussy.

The woman opposite me began, 'I would like to stroke your arm,' she said.

'Yes,' I said, with none of the hesitancy I'd felt when a man had asked the same thing in our first tantra week. I felt safe with her because she was a woman. It felt relaxing and uncomplicated to be there with her. Fun. I was not thinking about what I should or shouldn't be doing. I wasn't wondering if I was good enough. I was just enjoying myself.

When she stroked it I was surprised to feel my arm go up in goosebumps.

'I want to stroke your arm,' I said, and felt shy. I was so unused to knowing or voicing what I wanted. I usually handed over all responsibility to whoever I was with.

She nodded and smiled. I ran my fingers down her arm and she started to sigh. Her body quivered.

'I'm very sensitive,' she said. 'Sometimes my body reacts to tiny touches – is that OK?'

'Yes.' It was more than OK, it was incredible to see.

'I want to stroke your face,' she said.

I nodded. And she stroked my cheeks with such gentleness it was startling.

'I want to run my hand down your back,' she said, and I leant towards her so that she could. It felt divine.

I asked if I could do the same to her and was mesmerized by her quivering. She was the embodiment of everything I wanted to be – so free and unselfconscious.

She was a goddess. Shining eyes looked right at me.

'You are exquisitely beautiful,' she said to me. Tears pricked my eyes and I felt overcome by the love I felt coming from her.

'So are you,' I replied.

I felt shy of saying what I wanted to do next. What if it was too much and it would be rejected?

'I want to take off your top.' She nodded and asked if she could take mine off too.

'Yes!' I said, and then remembered I had no bra under my vest. As she pulled up my vest, I had hectic thoughts about the fact that I was now topless with a woman in a room full of people. What?! What did this mean?

'I want to kiss you,' I said.

She nodded, and I placed the softest kiss on her lips. I was used to kissing a face that was rough with stubble. This kiss felt smooth and . . . safe.

I found myself wanting to touch her breasts so I asked her if I could. She said yes and as I touched them I understood why men loved them so much. Breasts are beautiful! She let out a sigh as I touched her. 'Yes,' she sighed in what sounded like pleasure.

I was turned on . . . turned on by a woman. What did this mean? I'd never had an experience with a woman before. Did this mean I was gay? Bi? Queer? I let go of my thoughts and kept saying yes because that was what I wanted to say at that moment.

'How do you make your body do that?' I asked her, as we lay down and she quivered from head to toe.

'I do breathing exercises which awaken sexual energy.'

There had been a lot of talk of 'sexual energy' this week and I had no clue what it actually meant, but I watched in awe as her body shuddered. I felt that this woman was showing me the way, showing me what was possible.

'How did you get to be like this?' I asked her. 'You're so free . . . don't you have any hang ups about this stuff?'

'I used to have a lot of hang ups,' she smiled. 'I had an abusive childhood . . . I used to self-harm and I had an eating disorder. I hated my body. Then my mother died and something inside me said "enough". I was determined to reclaim my body and my sexuality and make it mine – not anyone else's – and here I am now.'

She was so beautiful – the most erotic woman I'd ever seen . . . so alive in her sexuality. She was like something out of *Dr. Quinn, Medicine Woman*, with shiny eyes that pierced my soul and a body that moved like water.

'You show me what a woman can be,' I said to her.

We were lying on a mattress on the floor chatting when a man we both knew asked if he could join us. We both looked at each other and agreed he could.

Jan kept telling us to breathe – explaining that when we are stressed our breathing becomes shallow and that we need to breathe to relax and to feel things, so I kept breathing, breathing, breathing . . . We started three-way kissing and it was funny and sexy and ridiculous and natural. I felt like this woman was my anchor, willing me on.

At some point during the kissing it felt like there was a magnet pulling my lips over this man's body, which looked like it had been carved out of oak. Soon we were three mouths and six hands, exploring. We were soft and slow and then passionate and then slow again . . . this woman knew how to say 'no' to anything she didn't like. It was said clearly and with love. I was learning from her.

At points it felt like I was being pulled by gravity into the ground, and at other times it felt like I was floating off the ground.

At one point the voice in my head said, *Look what you're doing! You can't do this! And don't touch his penis, you'll do it wrong! And stop kissing that woman! You're not gay!* – and then it floated away like a radio being turned down and my body kept doing what it wanted to do, almost of its own accord.

'Light dissolves shame,' Jan had said. 'We do not work together in groups because I am an advocate of polyamory, but because bringing our sexuality out into the open dissolves shame.'

10

Shame

There was no escaping shame when I got back to the real world. I dreamt that my pores were leaking rivers of mud and then, in some kind of biblical punishment, my shower got blocked and coffee grounds started coming up through the plug hole.

I was in shock at what this Irish Catholic middle-aged schoolgirl had done. Kissing women? And men? Giving hand jobs to men in Hawaiian shirts? Was I going to hell? What would my mother say?

The tantra WhatsApp group kept pinging as people shared their feelings about what they had experienced. People talked about shedding layers of shame and conditioning. They described their bodies as feeling new. Words like 'delicious' and 'melted' were used. Bodies were tingly and hearts bursting open. Hawaiian Santa felt like he was 'swimming in a sea of ecstasy'.

I wrote: *'I don't love my body. Feeling numb and teary.'*

Another woman wrote: *'Shame is the tax we pay on pleasure.'*

She sent a meme. It was a photo of an oily mound of bodies on satin sheets with the caption: 'What people think happens on a tantra retreat'. I scrolled down to find a second picture captioned: 'What actually happens'. The photo was a face crying.

———

The days after I came back, I doubled down on old numbing habits. I opened a can of Stella at 3 p.m., ordered noodles on Deliveroo and watched a Scandi murder. A woman had been cut in half at the waist and left in a car park.

One of the guys on the retreat had told me to watch *On Chesil Beach*, so when I'd had my fill of murdered women, I watched the film about a young couple's first night together as a married couple in 1962. Their ignorance around sex ends their marriage before it's even begun. I winced as I watched it. They were a product of wartime Britain, getting married before the sexual revolution, whereas I was brought up at a time when porn could be accessed as easily as a text message and sex was used to sell everything. But still, I related to their paralysis and awkwardness.

Why was that?

I listened to a *Goop* podcast episode with Esther Perel, a sex therapist. She believes we live in an age where we think we are past sexual shame but we are not. She said:

> For a long time we said that sex was sinful. Every civilization has tried to control sexuality, every religion . . . You need sex because without it you can't have society continue to exist, but you can't have too much of it or you can't control the people once they are immersed in this lustful pleasure. So, we grew up with a lot of silence around sexuality and today we would like to be able to talk about it openly, but it's very hard to talk suddenly, openly as an adult about everything you've learned to be so silent about . . . We carry guilt, we carry silence and we don't really know how to talk about it . . . For a long time, we said sex was sinful. Then when we tried to do away with religion, and we brought in the sexual revolution of the 60s, we replaced it with "sex is natural', which was a wonderful

thing to say in light of how much it had been condemned, and vilified. But on the other end, it's not natural. It's an art. It's cultivated, it's learned. It's an intelligence. It's a lot of things but it's not just something you know. And from that moment on, we have actually encouraged ignorance rather than the ability to learn about it, to talk about it from very early on.

I listened to this over and over again. It made me feel normal.

A few days later, I was in a post office returning a pair of jeans to The Outnet and the queue was long. An older man in front of me turned around and shook his head in frustration.

'We must be patient, I suppose,' he said.

I nodded. His white hair was trimmed into a cut that belonged on a schoolboy. He had a silver ring on his right hand.

'I'm buying stamps for my friend, there's a special collection out today. He only has a small post office near him, so I get them for him. Last month there was a set of Queen stamps and the woman in front of me took them all! So you have to get here early.'

'You're a good friend.'

He nodded. 'I like to do things for him.'

'That's nice.'

'We have known each other for fifty years. He is not well now. He is having an operation next week. So I do more. Get him food and bits.'

I nodded.

'If we were in today's world we would have been more than friends. I suppose we would have been . . .' He looked down at his Hush Puppies. 'Perhaps we would have been married,' he said.

'Oh, OK.'

'But my family doesn't know and his sister wouldn't allow it, so we never lived together. He is in South London. I visit once a week. He is older than me, he was eighty last year. He's not very well.'

His rheumy eyes were watery but he looked like a young boy with his satchel on his shoulder.

'We live in different times now,' he said.

'Yes,' I said.

'But it's too late for us.'

I felt my own eyes welling up.

'But you mustn't dwell. And I had good news last week. I have cancer – the man's kind – but it's the kind they say you die with rather than of.'

'Oh, OK, that's good,' I said.

'Must be patient,' he repeated.

He turned back around to face the front of the queue and I stood behind him, thinking of all the lives ruined by sexual shame. By sexual shame made into laws.

What a waste. The law was the crime, not their love.

Enough, enough, enough.

The thought of James or Ella being brought up in the same way was unbearable. The idea of them not being able to love whoever they wanted to love in whatever way they wanted to love them broke my heart. The idea of them depriving themselves of pleasure and touch, and of being ashamed of their bodies made me furious.

No, no, no. Enough. This is not how life should be.

Repressed. Ashamed. Scared. Ignorant. Unable to ask.

Enough.

What if my generation could be the last one to be ashamed of sex? Wouldn't that be amazing? So I had kissed a man and a woman. Touched men's penises in a room full of other people.

All of it had been done with love and respect, and it felt delicious. What could possibly be wrong with that? Really?

I was not going to be ashamed of sex any more.

Not going to be silent.

'You kissed a girl and you liked it!' said Daisy, when she came over. She was the first person I'd told about what happened during the week.

'I think this is so cool!' she said. 'You are on your way to being a master lover! A tantric goddess!'

She wanted to know if I was going to see any of them again and I said they all lived miles away.

'You're so cool,' she said.

'What do you mean?' I asked.

'If I was you, I'd be running after all of them.'

I told her I was going to see Jake from the festival. She opened her mouth and then closed it again. Then she said: 'Jake's a really nice guy, but . . . be careful.'

'What do you mean?'

'You know he sees other people.'

'Yes,' I said.

'Obviously, you do what feels good, love, and I'm all for you embracing your sexuality – you know that – but I'm just saying be careful. As a former slut, I don't think that physically and spiritually we are made to share our energy with lots of people. I thought I was fine, but I don't think it did me any good.'

'OK,' I said.

'I got sucked in by my shady narcissists who were trying to sell screwing around as spiritual enlightenment. I pretended to be OK but I wasn't really. I realized I couldn't do it, jumping around from one person to the next. I need the safety of a monogamous relationship. I want to go deep with one person.'

'Yeah, I know what you mean,' I lied. I didn't want to go deep with one person. Not at all. You go deep, you drown.

'But, love, you do whatever you want – you're older than I was when I was playing around, so you can probably handle it. Just be careful that you're not running away.'

Rachel had said this to me several times. *The Ethical Slut* warns of it too. It says that some people jump from partner to partner, always imagining the next partner will be the perfect one. These people 'may never stay with anyone long enough to discover the deeper intimacy and profound security that comes from confronting, struggling with, and conquering the hard parts of intimacy together.'

When I'd told Sarah about my interest in polyamory, she'd shot it down in one sentence: 'It's hard enough making one relationship work, how the fuck are you supposed to keep five going?' I didn't tell her about the retreat.

Rachel was more pragmatic about my recent sexcapades when I got the courage to give her some edited highlights: 'You spent a grand learning how to give a hand-job? I could have shown you that for the price of a cucumber.'

I went to see Jake anyway. He greeted me by his front door wearing a pair of multicoloured harem trousers and an open shirt that showed his tanned chest. His hair looked wild from a summer spent in fields. I felt prissy and suburban in my jeans, floral blouse and sandals.

He welcomed me into his studio-sized room at the top of the house and I sat on an armchair by a table piled with books while he made us herbal tea. I flicked through the books while he was in the kitchen. They were photo books of penises and vulvas. He came back in and we talked about the festivals he'd gone to. We went for a walk and held hands. I felt self-conscious holding hands. But I kept doing it. Then we went for tea and cake and he fed me some of his surprisingly tasty vegan flourless brownie. I cringed. I hated being fed. But I didn't say anything.

Despite all I'd done that summer, I was closing down, folding into my old, repressed ways.

We got back to his, hung out with his housemates and fell asleep together. We kissed a bit but I was feeling turned off. I apologized and he told me there was nothing to be sorry for.

When we woke up we kissed a bit more and he brought me tea in bed. He let me know that he had to leave at midday to meet a lover for brunch, then they were going to buy whips for a party that night. Again, I pretended this was normal to me and told him that it was OK, I had to head to a family thing.

The next day I was standing on the tiled floor of a Catholic church while my cousin and his wife offered their beloved baby to the priest.

The reception was in a bar built onto the side of the church. There was a buffet of white-bread sandwiches and quiches under cling film.

'Your turn next?' I felt a nudge by my side. It was my cousin in a suit holding his baby daughter, dwarfed in a long white dress and a little lacy headband. I smiled at her and told him she was gorgeous. Which she was.

'You going to make Mary a grandmother?' he persisted.

'Ha! I don't think so,' I said, grabbing a handful of crisps.

'How is your love life?' he asked.

'Uneventful,' I lied. I could not talk to my cousin about the joys of being an ethical slut with learner plates.

'Are you on the apps?' he asked.

'No,' I said.

'You've got to be in it to win it – it's a numbers game,' he said.

I nodded and moved to the other end of the table to load up on sausage rolls. My sister flinched as I lifted my arm to put more crisps on my paper plate.

'Are you a feminist or just lazy?'

I looked down at hairs poking out of my armpit and realized I hadn't shaved all summer. 'I dunno,' I said. 'Both?'

As we drove home, I wondered what Jake was up to with his mystery lover. I wondered what she looked like. I wondered if they were naked. I didn't feel jealous so much as out of my depth.

This was not my world – I was too far in the deep end.

We dropped mum off first. She wanted us to come in for a bit, so we went in and drank tea in front of the telly. A documentary about Leonard Cohen and his lover Marianne was on the BBC.

We watched as Leonard travelled the world bedding a different woman every day, while Marianne was left pining on a Greek island, both neglecting her son to the extent he ended up in an institution.

'That poor boy. Somebody always gets hurt,' said mum at the end. 'It's like that book about the Bloomsbury set – six couples always swapping around. You'd need to draw a map to keep on top of it. A lot of soul-searching and unhappiness.'

'Yeah, but I suppose they were exploring something new,' I said.

'I have no moral problem with it,' mum said. 'I just don't know how well it works in reality.'

'What was it like being alive in the Sixties?' I asked her.

'I don't know, I missed it. I was too busy being good.'

I felt like I had a choice. Be good like my mother or . . . explore a different way. Something unconventional and scary and potentially wonderful.

I believed wholeheartedly in the possibilities described in *The Ethical Slut* and the beauty I'd experienced at tantra. Both exuded the kind of love and goodness that my convent school was always telling us about, but failed to embody.

But did I have the courage to live that way?

I loved people who were not living a 'normal' life and yet I didn't have the guts to declare myself one of them. I was still, deep down, a Virgin Mary, trained to be 'good' and to fit in.

The next morning, I sent Jake a text saying that I had had a wonderful time but I was too conventional for him.

'I am saddened though not surprised by your choice,' he replied. 'Thank you for the time we spent together, I wish you joy and happiness in your life and most of all love. Big hugs, Jake xxx.'

It was the most beautiful and respectful text I'd ever received.

11

Unattached

'They only froze three eggs – not as many as I'd hoped,' said Rachel, when I went around for dinner.

'I'm sorry.'

'And I read another fucking article about fertility going off a cliff at thirty-five – I'm just sick of it – it's like no matter what we do, it's wrong. I didn't choose to be in this situation, I wanted to be with someone and have a family, but it just didn't happen. This idea that I prioritized my career – I didn't. Yes, I have a career, but I never put that before my relationships.'

'I know,' I said. She really hadn't. She always put people before work.

'I spoke to Kate the other day. I said I was tired and she basically laughed at me. Said I should try being awake all night with a teething baby. I get that she has two young kids and she can't sleep in, but she has help. Dave does everything for her and her parents are always over . . . I don't have any help with anything. I work on my own. I pay the mortgage on my own, I put up shelves on my own. When the boiler breaks it's me who needs to get it fixed, me who needs to get quotes for the fucking roof that's leaking again. I'm the one spending three hours on the phone to Virgin when the internet goes again, I'm the one who has to make dinner and empty the dishwasher and take the rubbish out . . . There's never anyone else doing that for me, it's just me. So yes, I'm tired. I'm tired of doing it all on my own all the time. She's tired because she got what she wanted – I'm tired because I didn't.'

We sat at her kitchen table, the night sky setting in the window behind her. I wished I could say something to make it better but I figured the best I could do was listen. I thought about the women's circle I'd gone to and how valuable it was to be able to talk without advice or reassurance.

'All my friends with kids make these comments about wishing they could lie in . . . and how they miss their single life. I'm sure they do, and I get it. But they're envying something they got to do already. Something they chose to move on from.

'I want what they have, but I can't go on about that because it's a downer and no guy will fancy me . . . and I hate that – like, there's this idea that life is fair and if you just make the right choices it'll all work out – but it isn't like that. It's all dumb fucking luck. And it's not just the kids, it's everything. I'm so tired of being alone. Like even when good things happen, I have nobody to tell.'

'You can tell me,' I said.

'I know, but I mean tiny things – yesterday a client paid after weeks of chasing, and I'm not going to call anyone to tell them that, but it would be nice to just have someone to tell over dinner and someone to say, that's great. I'm tired of being on my own. I'm tired of wishing I was still with Ben and remembering only the good bits of our relationship. I'm tired of thinking there's something wrong with me because this is my life. I keep going over all these versions of my life where I did things differently and made different decisions and ended up with what everyone else has . . . I thought that if you worked hard and did the right things, karma would look after you, but it just doesn't work like that. And if I don't meet someone – do I want a child enough to try to get pregnant using donor sperm? And how much money would I have to earn to put my child in nursery so that I could work to look after us both? And if I did it on my own, would every birthday and Christmas be like something is missing? Is it fair to bring a child up like that? Is it selfish?'

'I don't know,' I said. 'I don't think so, but I don't know.'

'And my aunt died.'

'You said. I'm sorry.'

'I was there when it happened, in the hospital.'

'I didn't realize.'

'Yeah, we were all in the hospital, her kids and me and my mum and my Uncle Tom . . . he climbed on the bed with her and was holding her as she went. And she did the death rattle – you know they say that, but it really happened, and my uncle just held her.'

She was crying now.

'And I thought, who's going to be there for me when I die? I know I have friends, but it's not the same – at moments like that. It isn't.'

I didn't say anything. Maybe she was right. With partners, commitments and promises were made. With friends there were no promises.

'Don't you ever think about things like that? Like, who's going to look after you when you're old?' she asked me.

'Not really,' I said. 'I can't see past dinner. And I still think I'm fifteen.' I laughed, but the joke felt flimsy. When *was* I going to grow up? Start thinking about these things?

'But don't you ever feel that you'd like someone around now? Don't you ever wish you had someone to tell stuff to, or someone to make you a cup of tea in the morning?'

I thought about it.

'I dunno, I guess I tell my mum and sister things . . .' I'd never had anyone make me tea in the morning – or coffee. The thought of that little act of kindness made me squirm – I didn't know why.

'And don't you want to leave something of you behind? Like what if you die and that really is it? There's nothing left of you?'

'That would be OK with me.'

'But would it?'

'Yes, it really would.'

I could see her straining to understand me as much as I was straining to understand her.

'I really don't think about things like that,' I said. 'I don't know why, but I don't.'

I offered to stay over. I lay next to her as she cried. In the morning I brought her a cup of tea in bed.

On the train home I thought about Rachel's hunger for a family and my own lack of hunger.

'I like my own space; I like to have chats with people and then go home,' I'd said to her when she questioned me on how I kept doing things on my own.

'And is that really enough for you?' she'd asked.

'Yes,' I said.

But I doubted myself. If I kept going like this, would I end up dying alone? Would my body be found three weeks after my death? Would this independence I prided myself on turn out to be a sham?

Daisy had told me there was a word for people like me – we were 'avoidant'. When I got back from Rachel's I dug out the book she had given me, with the annoying heart-magnet cover. On the front of the book was an endorsement from John Gray, author of *Men Are from Mars, Women Are from Venus*. He declared it to be 'a groundbreaking book that redefines what it means to be in a relationship'.

I'd read *Men Are from Mars* years ago. I couldn't remember what it said beyond men wanting to retreat into a cave and women wanting to talk a lot. When I read it I wanted to be the man.

Attached: The new science of adult attachment and how it can help you find – and keep – love by Dr. Amir Levine and Rachel S. F. Heller, M. A. was published in 2011 but its terminology was becoming widespread on social media, with people talking about their attachment styles in the same way we talk about our star signs.

Attachment theory is based on the fact that we are all biologically programmed to be in close relationships with our caregivers as infants. We are hardwired to bond with other people because in our infancy days our physical survival depended on it. The need to be near someone special is so important that the brain has a biological mechanism, called the 'attachment system', that consists of emotions and behaviours that ensure we stay close to our loved ones.

But while we all have this need for attachment, the way we show it differs.

'Secure' people feel comfortable with intimacy and are usually warm and loving. They are happy with space, and also happy with togetherness. They don't blow hot and cold. 'Anxious' people, on the other hand, crave intimacy and are often preoccupied with their relationships but tend to worry that their partner doesn't love them back or is going to leave. Finally, 'avoidant' people equate intimacy with a loss of independence and are always trying to keep their distance from others. As I read on, it became clear that I was an avoidant, but just to be sure, I did a quiz that asked readers to tick the statements that were true for us:

- I find that I can bounce back quickly after a break-up. It's weird how I can just put someone out of my mind. *True.*
- My independence is more important than my relationships. *True.*
- I prefer not to share my innermost feelings with my partner. *True. People can hurt you and laugh at you and tell you that your innermost feelings are stupid and wrong. Why would you risk that?*
- I sometimes feel angry or annoyed with my partner without knowing why. *True.*
- I prefer casual sex with uncommitted partners to intense sex with one person. *Probably true.*
- It makes me nervous when my partner gets too close. *True.*
- I hate feeling the other person depending on me. *True true true.*

As I ticked, I noticed I got a kick out of my independence. There was a teenage bravado to it: see, I don't care, you can't hurt me! I don't need you!

My pride crumbled as I read the 'deactivating strategies' avoidants use to keep people at a distance, which include:

- Focusing on imperfections in your partner: the way he talks, dresses etc. *Oh. I do that with every man I've ever even thought about getting involved with.*
- Pining after an ex or waiting for The One. *I have been thinking about the Greek a lot . . .*

- Not saying 'I love you'– while implying you do have feelings for them. *Yeah, but I'd said 'I love you' once and then he thought that meant we were going to be together for ever, so I took it back.*
- Pulling away when it's going well (e.g. not calling after an intimate date). *Yeah, but why does everyone want to be on the phone all the time? I'm done with all these messages! And calls. Why can't people back off?*
- Forming impossible relationships, such as with married men. *Or men in Greece?*
- Avoiding physical closeness – for example, not wanting to share the same bed, not wanting to have sex, walking several strides ahead of your partner. *OK, well, I'm a fast walker. So what?*
- Keeping secrets and keeping things foggy – to maintain your feeling of independence. *Yes.*

I had never seen my behaviour so clearly mapped out before.

This was the missing piece of the puzzle. This was why I was the way I was in relationships. But instead of feeling peace about it, I felt awful.

There was no teenage bravado now: I was a bitch.

The book concludes that avoidants treat the person closest to them the worst. They respond to other people's feelings like they are in a court of law rather than really understanding their point of view. They say things to devalue their partner. They don't pick up on what their partner is feeling because they are too wrapped up in themselves. They blame anxious people for being jealous and needy and make the anxious partner feel constantly rejected. They look down on people with needs, accusing them of being weak and needy. In short, we – I – treat our lovers like they're the enemy.

'I don't understand why anyone would want to go near an avoidant,' I said to Daisy. 'We're awful.'

'People like you are crack for people like me,' she said.

'Why? What type are you?' I asked, but I knew the answer: she was anxious.

When she met someone, she texted them fifteen times a day, lost in the excitement of this new love. The book explains how for people with anxious attachment the priority is to stay connected, even if the relationship is no good for them.

'We're hooked on the drama. The chase feels like love to us even though it isn't,' said Daisy. 'And maybe, deep down, there's a bit of me that doesn't feel like I deserve love, which is why I go after people that will never give it to me.'

'That's sad,' I said.

'I'm looking for love to save me,' she continued. 'I'm looking for the love I didn't get as a child, but then I go for these guys who won't offer it to me, which confirms how I felt in the beginning – crap and unloveable.'

I was in awe of how clearly she saw herself.

'Does knowing all this stop you from going for the wrong people?' I asked.

'No! But maybe one day it will,' she laughed.

'So why do avoidants like me end up with people like you?'

'You're attracted to us because we carry all the vulnerability; we do all the worrying so you can play it cool,' she said.

'Oh.'

'And, deep down, you like the attention.'

That was true. I wanted to be wanted, but only when I wanted it, and then I wanted people to back off.

'And also, there's a theory that people who avoid closeness are deep down afraid of being abandoned. And people who fear abandonment – like me – are really scared of engulfment, which is why we always go for partners who are emotionally unavailable – in reality, we are scared of getting too close to someone. Otherwise, we wouldn't keep picking the people we do.'

God, this was a minefield.

I'd never heard the word 'engulfment' before.

I probably was scared of being abandoned.

I remembered as a kid thinking that after every summer holiday my friends would not want to be my friends any more. They'd have gone off and done exciting things that summer and when they came back to school, all tanned from foreign adventures and new beach buddies, they'd ditch me. Pretend they didn't even know me.

It never happened, but every year I expected it to and every year I was braced for pretending not to care. That was my defence mechanism: to pretend not to care. Maybe I'd pretended so much I now believed it.

I said that to Daisy.

'You might be a fearful avoidant,' she said.

'What's that?'

'It's when you are anxious *and* avoidant. The worst of both worlds.'

'Great.'

'Or you could be a love anorexic,' said Daisy.

I rolled my eyes at the jargon. All these online quizzes to find out your love language, attachment style . . . Was any of it doing us any good? Still, I took the bait. 'What's that?'

'It's someone who starves themselves of love and affection.'

I remembered going on a date with a man who told me that I fetishized aloneness. He also thought I fetishized sleep and work. I thought he fetishized the word fetishize. Other than that, he was a nice guy, smart and funny. But I didn't want to see him again. He was shorter than me and I didn't like his jacket.

I wondered what he was up to now.

Had he got married? Fallen in love with a person who fetishized togetherness? He was buying a flat at the time. I wondered if he had climbed the property ladder . . . I wondered what life would have been like if I'd agreed to another date. I could have led a whole different life, a 'normal', home-owning-couple life, with savings. (What did it say about me that the main value I could see in partnerships was financial?)

Anyway, it didn't matter. I only saw him once.

I had dismissed him, and others, so quickly and easily. Too tall, too short, too quiet, too loud, too into work, not ambitious enough . . . I was the Goldilocks of dating, when I could be bothered to do it.

'The book says that nobody will be good enough for me because I keep finding faults,' I said to Daisy. 'But how do I know the difference between when someone really *isn't* right for me and when they might be right but I'm just scared of being close?'

'That's the million-dollar question,' she said.

'And is it saying I have to be in a couple to be a happy human being? Or is it talking about relationships in general, like friends?'

'I think friends count as relationships,' said Daisy.

'But all the anecdotes are romantic and there's a heart on the cover. I think it's saying you have to be in a couple.'

'I don't know . . .'

'And I don't understand what you're supposed to do about the way you are.' And as I said it, I realized I felt quite desperate about this. 'So now I know I'm avoidant – what do I *do*? How can I be different from the way I am?'

'Doesn't the book say that we should go out with secure people and model their behaviour?'

'I don't know, I haven't got that far yet. I'm stuck on the bit that's telling me what a bitch I am.'

'It's been a few years since I read it, but I think it says that we have to get good at asking for what we need – so I need to explain to people that I like to speak every day and get replies to my texts. And maybe for you it's about asking people for space . . . Have you heard from the Greek, by the way?' she asked.

'Yeah, we spoke last week. He just got a new mattress . . .' I don't know why I told her that, but I liked that he'd told me that.

'He says he loves me at the end of calls,' I added.

'Do you say it back?'

'No. What about you? Are you still on Bumble?' I asked.

'Yeah, but I'm going to delete it. I need to be single for a while.'

She'd said this before.

'The thing is,' she continued, 'I keep going out with guys who don't commit and who use me as some kind of ego boost but I'm just as bad. I'm using these guys just as much as they're using me. They're using me for sex or attention or whatever, and I'm using them so that I never have to be alone.

'It's never really about them at all,' she continued. 'And that's not right.'

'Wow,' I said. 'You see it all so clearly. And do you think you can do that – be on your own?'

'I've started therapy again,' she said. 'And this job is going well, so yeah, maybe . . .'

'That sounds really good. Liquorice, rose or turmeric?' I asked, opening the cupboard and looking at the rainbow of herbal-tea boxes.

'Let's do a cocktail – liquorice and rose. What's the message?' she asked.

I looked at the labels attached to the teabags. ' "The art of happiness serves all" . . . and "Sing from your heart".'

'They're so vague now.'

'Weren't they always?'

'No – I once left a job based on a Yogi Tea message.'

'What did it say?'

'I can't remember.'

As we drank our tea, I asked Daisy, 'Do you think I'm cold?' There was a pause.

'No . . .' – another pause – '. . . but I think you are defensive in this area . . . and you can be quite intimidating,' said Daisy.

I couldn't imagine being intimidating to anyone.

'I think you give off the vibe that you don't need anyone.'

I'd heard that before.

'And you're not very patient with people who aren't—'

'Aren't what?' I interrupted.

'Articulate.'

'Oh. OK . . .'

'I'm not trying to be harsh, love. I just want you to know how you come off . . . maybe to men.'

'OK.'

'But the right guy will see through all that stuff. I can totally picture him . . . he has very shiny shoes and smells good and is wearing a scarf from – what's that shop you like? The old one?'

'Liberty?'

'Yeah, he's wearing a scarf from Liberty, and he's very tall . . .'

'Nice.' I was smiling now.

'He's divorced because he got married too young, and he has a daughter . . .'

'Right.'

'She's at university – and she really likes you.'

'Where do I meet this nice-smelling unicorn?'

'Not on the apps – he's too old-fashioned for that. You meet by chance when you're out one night seeing a friend in a place you don't normally go to . . . somewhere businessy.'

'Oh, OK.'

'You aren't expecting to meet anyone, you're deep in chat with your friend so you're glowing, and then at the bar you strike up conversation with this guy . . . and the fireworks start to fizz.'

'Right . . .'

'You exchange numbers and he sends you a message a few days later and says he needs a plus one for something fancy . . .'

'Ooh.'

'There's just one issue.'

'What is it?'

'His sister is a bitch.'

I laughed.

'She makes candles and lives in Chiswick.'

'Of course she does.'

I fell asleep thinking of a man with shiny shoes, and while in some fairy-tale way it was a comforting thing to think about, it also made me feel stressed and powerless.

It brought me back to that old feeling that there was something missing from my life and that the answer came in the form of a man I had not yet met and may never meet – and until I did meet him, I would be unfinished, incomplete, lacking.

It bothered me that *Attached* seemed to be saying the

exact opposite of the single-positivity movement. Books like *Spinster* and *The Unexpected Joy of Being Single* made me feel empowered because they told me that I didn't need to be with someone, that I was enough as I was, that I had a freedom and autonomy that generations of women had fought for. *The Ethical Slut* told me I could take this autonomy and have gorgeous, loving, respectful sex too.

Attached was making me feel like all this independence and sexual exploration was a way of running away – and that one day I'd regret it.

12

Domestic Bliss

James ran towards me with his arms open.

I let go of my bag and he jumped up and I caught him. All my life I'd been waiting for a romantic airport meeting, and finally it had happened.

'MARIAAAAAANNE!' – he turned back to Gemma – 'Marianne is here!' – and then turned back to me again. 'Mummy parked outside and I got a new car and it's yellow and mummy says you are staying with us for a week and I got a new tractor and Maureen lets me play with her puppy—'

'Oh my god! So much news!' I squeezed and lifted him and kissed his shiny cheeks.

He wriggled and I lowered him to the floor. He shoved his open hand in front of me.

'Look, it's yellow!' he said of the toy car sitting in his perfect palm.

'I love it!' I said.

'I got a new tractor too and a trailer but that's in the car. And I've left a present in your bed.'

'Thank you!'

'It's a surprise.'

'Exciting!'

'It's a car but you can't keep it, it's just to borrow.'

'So what's the surprise?'

'What car it is.'

'I've never seen him do that before,' said Gemma, moving in for a hug.

'What?'

'Run into someone's arms like that.'

I was chuffed.

I hugged her and smelled her familiar perfume and kissed her cheek too.

'I've missed you,' I said.

As soon as we got outside I smelled Irish turf burning. My shoulders dropped.

'It smells like home,' I said.

'God, this is so beautiful.'

I'd seen Gemma's house during various stages of the renovations but this was the first time I'd seen it finished. She and her husband had restored an old cottage with such care it felt like stepping into a painting.

Everywhere I looked was beauty. A wild garden visible through French doors off the kitchen, the old-fashioned stove with copper pots simmering, a marble fireplace in the living room. It was like a work of art.

Alex was making a roast chicken. We hugged and he offered me a glass of wine, and, as I sat down at the large wooden dining table with flowers on it, James ran into the kitchen to show me more cars and Lego.

While I played with him, Gemma helped Alex with lunch. I glanced over and saw them move around the kitchen together. Gemma touched Alex on the back, to signal her desire to get to the cutlery. She handed him a tea-cloth as he opened the oven. It was a silent dance of two bodies who were used to working as a team.

Eighties music was playing from the speakers and I drank my wine and smiled.

This is a beautiful life, I thought.

After we'd finished eating the kind of meal that belonged in a Sunday supplement magazine, Alex cleared the table and loaded the dishwasher while Gemma and I stayed chatting and drinking wine.

'Does he always do that?' I asked Gemma.

'Do what?'

I pointed to Alex, who was unloading the dishwasher after we'd spent two hours talking.

She smiled. 'Of course, we both do it.'

It blew my mind to see a man unload a dishwasher. It also blew my mind to see him roasting a chicken and offering to take James for a run around in the park.

My therapist had said that I had an old-fashioned view of relationships and family life. I'd been brought up in a family where dad went out to work and mum stayed home. Growing up, the only thing dad knew how to work in the kitchen was the toaster, which he used to light his cigars. Apparently, things had moved on.

It rained that evening so we stayed home, moving to the living room to watch *Fantastic Mr. Fox*. I sat on an old leather armchair while Gemma and Alex had the sofa, Gemma's legs stretched out on top of Alex's. James was sitting on a big cushion by their feet. They were the picture of happiness. Peace and easy, familial love.

Why did I spend so much time running from this?

I heard knocking and turned over to ignore it. James was leaning against my bed

My eyes felt gritty.

'It's time to get up!' he said. 'Mummy told me I had to wait until eight and it's eight now.'

'OK.' My head was pounding and I kept my eyes closed.

'Will you play cars with me?' James was asking.

'Can I have my coffee first?' I said, this time looking at him and his perfect face.

'And then we'll play cars after?'

'Yes,' I said. I wanted to lie in bed all day. If I was at home with a hangover like this I would lie in bed all day.

The kitchen was too bright. 'Morning,' I said to Gemma. 'What time were you up?'

'About six.'

'How do you do it?'

'You get used to it.'

I had coffee and toast. James stayed by my side.

'Can we play cars now?'

I lay on the floor of the living room while he explained the rules. I wasn't listening.

'You're not listening!' he said.

'I am!' I said.

For about three millennia we wheeled the cars around the carpet. There were breakdowns. Crashes. The police were called at a couple of points, and the fire brigade. Sirens were mimicked and very serious emergencies – which were narrated with an 'Oh NO!' from James – dealt with.

I wanted to take ten paracetamol and crawl behind the sofa.

'Let's play football!'

'It looks like it might rain,' I said.

'Pleeeeease.'

'Can I have a shower first?' I said.

When I came out, James was waiting by the door to the bathroom.

He explained the rules.

I wasn't listening.

'You're not listening!' he said.

'I am!' I said.

We kicked the ball back and forth for five millennia. Kick. Kick. Kick. Kick. I entered an altered state through boredom, tiredness and hungoverness. Moodiness descended . . . a moodiness that reminded me of childhood. I felt trapped, like I had on Sunday afternoons when everyone was in a bad mood and there was nowhere to go. When family life felt like a prison sentence.

The sky was heavy and it was going to rain any second.

'You cheated!' James shouted.

'How was I cheating?' I asked.

'You went over the line.'

'What line?'

'The line!' he said, drawing an imaginary line on the grass.

'You didn't tell me about the line!' I said.

'I did!'

'You didn't!'

He crossed his arms and jutted his bottom lip out and I did the same right back.

'No!' he said, showing excellent boundaries.

'No what?'

'Just no!'

'Fine – if you don't want to play any more we don't have to,' I said.

'I DO want to play but you can't go over THE LINE.'

He stomped his foot on the grass and jutted his lip out even more.

I stomped my foot on the grass too and stuck out my tongue.

Then I realized that I was meant to be the adult.

After that I surrendered.

If James wanted to play football, we played football. If he wanted to go on an 'avventure', we went on one. If he wanted to orchestrate a complicated scenario in which the fire truck was not allowed to go in the direction it was going because there had been a crash and we had to create a new route . . . well, then we created a new route.

And then something happened.

On the flip side of the resistance, I discovered serenity. I was no longer in control of my time. My life, my thoughts, weren't that important at all. He couldn't give a shit whether I wrote a book or replied to that email. He just wanted me here, with him, now. And it was a relief; a relief for it not to be all about me.

I fell into a James trance, following him wherever he wanted to take me – whether that was kicking a ball or walking up the road or playing tractors. Every morning would start with him coming into my room and saying that mum said it was OK for him to wake me. I told him that he was the best thing to see at the start of any day. And he was.

One day James leant up against the bed and watched me put on my make-up.

'My mummy has that,' he says, pointing to a Benefit blusher. 'But she has a brush in the box.'

'I had a brush too but I lost it, so now I use this big one.'

'You need to look after your things better,' said James.

'I do. That's true,' I said.

'Can I have some?' he asked, looking at me with his face that looked like the sun.

I ran the brush over his cheeks and wished it was cleaner for his perfect, plump skin. He looked in the mirror and turned his head.

'It's sparkly,' he said.

'Yeah, it is a bit. You're ready to go to a party now.'

'We had a party and we had burgers.'

'Nice. Your mum makes great burgers.'

'On the barbecue.'

'Yum.'

'It's broken,' he said when I opened up the eyeshadow that had smashed into brown shards.

'I know. I should get a new one.'

He looked at the mucky make-up and then at me.

'You look after your friends instead of your things,' he announced.

I looked at him. Stunned. It was one of the nicest things anyone had ever said to me.

Later that day we all went for a walk. James wanted to keep stopping to pick up leaves and poke sticks at the grass, but I was rushing us home. After about ten minutes James stood still.

'Come on, we're almost home,' I lied.

'No.'

'James, it's not much longer,' I said, coaxing.

'No,' he said again, this time making his point heard by lying down on the path. I started walking on, hoping he'd follow me. He didn't. I walked back to him. There was only one option.

I lay down next to him.

We kept looking in silence for a while.

'That cloud looks like a cow,' James said, pointing.

'Oh yeah, it does,' I replied, and it really did. 'That one looks a bit like a pig,' I said, pointing to another one.

'No, it doesn't!' he giggled.

'Marianne,' he said, a while later.

'Yes, James.'

'I love you.'

'I love you, too.'

On the final night James asked if I could do bath time with him. Afterwards, I wrapped him in a hot-pink towel hanging behind the bathroom door. I read him a story, and before I turned out the light I stood by the door, drinking him in, tucked under the white duvet, looking like a dream wrapped in a cloud.

'I can't believe the pink towel is still going,' I said to Gemma, back in the kitchen.

We had bought it together when we were working in newspapers in Dublin, and G was dreaming of buying a cottage near where she grew up. TK Maxx had just opened and we were making regular pilgrimages to furnish this would-be country dwelling. One weekend, G picked up the giant, hot-pink towel.

'Would it look good in the cottage?' she'd asked.

'Definitely,' I said.

'You don't think it's too over the top?'

'No, it's perfect.'

There was just one problem.

'What happens when I get a boyfriend and he comes to stay? How will he feel about having to use a pink towel?'

For about ten minutes we stood in the shop having a serious conversation about whether the boyfriend she did not yet have would have an objection to towels she had not yet bought for a house that she did not own.

We burst out laughing.

She bought the towels.

She bought the cottage.

She got the boyfriend.

They got married, and a couple of years later they had a baby boy whom I loved more than I could imagine possible.

'I love him so much that when I'm at home I sometimes crave him, like literally crave him,' I said to Gemma, who was on the sofa, rubbing cream into her legs.

'He loves you too,' she said.

'You're such a good mum,' I told her.

'I don't know about that. He's a good child, we got lucky.'

'No, I think you're making him what he is,' I said.

She really was an exceptional mother. Sarah too. I didn't know how they knew how to do it . . . or how they poured so much love and energy into everyone around them – kids, partners, colleagues, me.

'You and Alex are happy together, aren't you?' I asked.

'There's no one else I'd rather fight with,' she smiled.

She asked if I wanted to keep seeing any of the men I'd met.

'I don't know. I don't think I'm cut out for all that.'

'All what?'

'Being in a couple.'

'Of course you are, if that's what you want. And if you don't, that's fine too.'

I appreciated her saying that. That whatever I did was fine. 'I'm always seeing guys for you,' she said. 'Tall, twinkly, smiley ones . . .' I smiled at how well she knew me.

'And are you sure you don't want kids?' asked Gemma. 'You don't mind me asking, do you? Whatever you do is great, but I feel like I wouldn't be a good friend if I didn't ask.'

'I know. I worry I'll regret it, but right now I can't make myself want something I don't.' I paused. 'I love James, and if anything happened to you I'd take him in a heartbeat and I'm sure it would be the best thing to ever happen to me . . . but I don't think I want my own.'

Why *was* that?

I loved kids.

I had spent so much time with James when he was a baby, I was dubbed his 'second mother'. I loved the absolute rightness of holding him on my hip. The perfect plumpness of his flawless skin. His tiny tiny fingernails . . . I'd look into his crystal eyes and think wow, wow, wow, this is a miracle. This little being is a miracle. As he grew up, I'd stand by his bedroom door watching him sleep, his brown limbs flung out of the white duvet, his blonde hair stuck in sweaty clumps on his forehead, and I'd yearn to climb into his head and watch his dreams. I didn't just love him, I loved who I was when I was with him.

I loved that being with him stopped the constant analysis in my head. I stopped being neurotic and was plugged into another life that was more important than mine. I loved that something primal kicked in and I knew what to do with him.

I had a purpose. I was needed. Of use.

So why wasn't I having my own? Was it just because I hadn't met the right guy? Or had I met perfectly right guys but was just too scared to give it a chance?

I had associated relationships – particularly romantic ones – with giving myself up completely. I had thought it would make me stop as a person, that I would lose myself.

My therapist had asked me to think about examples of happy relationships. At the time, Barack and Michelle Obama had sprung to mind.

'What do you admire about that relationship?' my therapist had asked.

'I imagine that they challenge and support each other, and that they communicate, so unsaid stuff doesn't build up . . . and that they have fun together.'

'And what do you think it would feel like to be in a relation-ship like that?' she'd asked.

'Um . . . safe and inspiring.'

But now I was really seeing a happy relationship, this time up close. I thought of Gemma describing how anytime she put her head on Alex's chest, she fell into a deep sleep. Being with him calmed her like nothing else did.

It was not a fairy tale. It was not perfect. But it was real and it looked like a nice place to be.

On the plane home I read the rest of *Attached*.

It explains that there is an evolutionary reason for me being the way I was. Historically, in very harsh environments where large numbers died from hunger, disease or natural disasters, it made sense not to get too attached. If loved ones died, you needed to move on quickly and not fall apart – hence the avoidant style. In other environments, the best survival chance might come from being hypervigilant about keeping the people they loved close – which was how anxious attach-ers were born. Finally, in peaceful places, intimate bonds were safe on all sides . . . which led to the secure attachment style.

I imagined my forefathers up an icy mountain with a woolly mammoth coming to get them and my great-great-grandfather being OK when his family was wiped out. He'd keep going . . .

But I wasn't living up a mountain. My family was not about to be wiped out. And the book argues that by constantly going it alone, the person I was hurting most was myself. It shares a study of women who were told they were going to be given an electric shock. They were told this to elicit a stress response in the brain. When the women were holding some-one's hand as they were given the news, the stress response was lower than when they were on their own. When they were holding their husbands' hands it was lower still. When they were holding their husbands' hands and had reported it to be a happy marriage, the stress was barely perceptible.

Reading this made me sad. I had spent my life getting electric shocks on my own.

They describe something called the 'Dependency Paradox', which describes the fact that when you bond securely with another human, you are, perhaps counterintuitively, more independent and brave in forging your own path.

The authors say: 'Our partners powerfully affect our ability to thrive in the world. There is no way around that. Not only do they influence how we feel about ourselves but also the degree to which we believe in ourselves and whether we will attempt to achieve our hopes and dreams.'

Avoidants describe themselves as free spirits, but it's all an act, according to the book. Our avoidance is a defence strategy that drops as soon as there is a disaster. If we get cancer or lose our house, we cling to others like an anxious person.

The book also says that by avoiding partnership, we prevent ourselves from experiencing one of the most beautiful things in life: the joy of being part of something bigger than ourselves. They caution that an avoidant's need to be self-reliant can involve too much focus on the self. Which was the story of my life.

Maybe I'd got everything wrong. Maybe I *did* want love? A partnership? Maybe even a family?

13

Intimacy

Jan was in a red outfit and her Madonna mic, looking at me solemnly standing in front of a room full of people.

'Do you take this man to have and to hold, to love and to cherish?'

I looked at the slight, blonde man with pink cheeks and a red T-shirt.

'I do,' I said, hot with self-consciousness.

She turned to him: 'And do you take this woman to have and to hold, to love and to cherish?'

'I do,' he said, looking down at his feet.

'I now pronounce you man and wife . . . for the next twenty-four hours!' said Jan, and moved on to the couple standing next to us, and repeated the procedure.

In all, eight couples were married that day. We were to arrange how we wanted to spend the time – whether we would be a tied-at-the-hip couple, or a free-to-roam pair.

'Well,' I said, trying to be perky. 'Hello, husband!'

'Hello, wife!' he said, using the same tone.

I didn't know what to say next. Neither did he. We both looked at our feet.

'So, have you been married before?' I asked him.

'No – you're my first wife,' he said.

'You're my first husband.'

We laughed nervously.

'Um, so shall we go for lunch?' he said.

We queued for jacket potatoes and salads and I talked nervously about not liking mushrooms and how mushrooms kept appearing in everything. I was telling him that I liked the look of mushrooms and wanted to like the taste of them, but didn't. I was talking too fast and boring myself. He looked into the middle distance. Blank.

'Sorry,' he said. 'My blood sugar gets low and I find it hard to concentrate when I'm hungry.'

We stood in line silently. I felt stressed. I didn't really know this man and he didn't know me. And now we were attached to each other for the rest of the day and night. What was I meant to do? How was I meant to behave?

After coming home from seeing Gemma in Ireland I had fallen into a hole. Daisy had gone away on a month-long yoga retreat, Sarah was busy with work and family, and Rachel was in Germany for work.

Seeing a happy family up close had made me see how lonely my life could be. As the weeks passed in the normal blur of work and sleep and eating cheese on toast, the freedom I so craved started to feel like emptiness.

I kept thinking of Rachel telling me I was running away from intimacy. And so I signed up to another Jan Day retreat called 'Intimacy, Authentic Relating & Love'. It gave participants the opportunity to get 'married' to experience how we felt when faced with commitment and closeness to another – even just for a day and a night.

We piled up our plates and found somewhere to sit together, and I fought the urge to fill the silence with inane chat as he ate. After a few mouthfuls he said, 'Thank you for giving me time – I was hungry. I feel better now.' I liked the way he said it. It was simple and clear. It made me feel relaxed to know what was going on with him. He wasn't being quiet because he hated me or because I was boring him with my mushroom chat – he just needed to eat. I realized how much misunderstanding had been spared by this simple communication and it made me realize how rarely I told people what was going on with me. I kept everything to myself.

We talked about normal stuff – where he was from, why he'd come to the retreat, how he was finding it. He seemed to avoid eye contact, mostly looking at his plate or the wall, which I found off-putting at first, but then a relief. He wasn't one of those over-the-top eye-gazers.

After we'd finished, I looked at the clock. We had half an hour left until we went back into sessions. I had wanted to wash my hair during lunch but I worried that that would feel like I was abandoning him. Was it selfish to go wash my hair when I'd just got married? Would it be running away? Did he want to spend the whole lunch break together? Would it be better to stay here with him?

I decided it was. Relationships mean compromise and that meant not washing my hair. But then I realized that was ridiculous.

'Do you mind if I go and wash my hair?' I asked.

'Of course I don't mind,' he said.

'What do you need from a relationship? And what are your wants?' Jan asked through her mic. 'And do you know the difference between your needs and your wants?'

The people around me were scribbling in their journals.

Needs and Wants, I wrote and underlined. My pen hovered over the paper.

Needs and Wants.

Needs and wants . . .

When we'd started again after lunch I looked around the

room for my husband and was relieved that he was sitting next to another woman and talking to her. Good, I thought, he's OK. I don't need to look after him. I can do my own thing.

Needs and wants.

I didn't know what my needs and wants were.

I mean, I needed food and oxygen and sleep, and surely that was it? I didn't need anything else.

I wrote: *I need sex and support and love.* But I hated the way that felt. I didn't *need* any of these things. I mean, they would be nice – to a point – but I didn't need them.

I crossed them out.

That felt better.

OK – wants.

Wants . . . Wants. Wants. Wants. Wants.

I wanted to have money and nice clothes and go travelling and have my own house. I wanted to keep writing and do well, and . . . just as my mind was going off into a lovely daydream, I realized nothing I was thinking about was connected with relationships.

OK. So, what did I want from a relationship?

Straight away I shut myself down with the phrase 'I want doesn't get' – which we heard every day from the nuns at school.

Come on, Marianne. Try. What do you want?

I want to be listened to. As I wrote that I felt it to be true. I really did want to be listened to. I rarely felt listened to . . . I was usually the one doing the listening.

And I want space. Yes. Also true.

And I want beautiful, mind-blowing, no hang-ups sex. Yes! I really did want that.

And I want them to go away when I want them to . . .

So that's mind-blowing sex, good listening and someone who will vanish. Was it OK that the main thing I wanted in relationships was space? I looked at my husband across the room, scribbling next to the other woman. Was it strange that I was happy he was with another woman?

I went back to my needs. Just as I did, Jan asked the group how many people had difficulty acknowledging their needs? A few hands went up. She said that people often say they don't have needs because they worry that having needs makes you needy – but we all have basic human needs; we need to be understood, to have autonomy, to love, we need to be able to trust and be responded to.

She explained that if you pretended that you had no needs for sex, affection or emotional support, you were lying to yourself, and you would wind up trying to get your needs met by indirect methods that didn't work very well.

Oh.

She then asked us what made us feel safe.

I wrote a list: *My mum, my bed, television, being in Ireland, Boxing Day* – oh the bliss of Boxing Day when everything is closed and nobody wants anything from you – *tea, toast, coffee shops, chocolate.*

Then I realized she meant what made us feel safe in relationships.

I wrote a new list: *Having space. Not feeling under pressure. People asking if I'm OK. People listening to me. People who don't get angry. Honesty. People doing what they say they'll do.*

Jan asked us to describe a vision of how we'd like to be in relationships. 'Write it in the present tense, as if it's already happening.'

More scribbling in the notebooks of everyone around me.

HOW I WANT TO BE IN A RELATIONSHIP.

I am a vibrant, powerful, sexual woman, I wrote.

I am relaxed, I have fun, I am spontaneous and playful and open to people and I am light and laugh and dance with life.

I DANCE WITH LIFE. I underlined that. I liked it.

I allow myself joy and pleasure and have no shame.

I keep my freedom.

I do not isolate.

I state my needs in a relationship – I communicate clearly and honestly.

I am vulnerable and gentle.

People read out their vision of relationships. Most of them talked in terms of 'we'.

'We live by the beach', 'We travel all the time', 'We have amazing sex'.

There was no 'we' in my list. Just me, me, me.

Was that the problem?

My husband and I avoided each other during the afternoon tea break. At least I knew I was avoiding him, and I'm pretty sure he was avoiding me. When we came back into the workshop room, I saw him sitting alone and I went up to him.

'Are you OK?' I asked.

'Yes,' he said. 'Are you?'

'Yes. Is it OK to sit next to you?' I asked and he said of course, but I had a strong feeling that he didn't want me to. Was that in my imagination or was it true? While I'd felt relieved that he was sitting next to another woman after lunch, that relief had turned into something else, something that was bugging me . . . something that felt like rejection. Why didn't he want to sit next to me? Why wasn't he looking for me? I wanted him to want to be near me.

We sat in a circle as Jan explained what intimacy was.

'To be intimate is to be known, to see and be seen, fully. It is to be naked, whether our clothes are on or off.' She explained that we could be intimate without being sexual and we could be sexual without being intimate. When the two are combined, something transformational happens: 'We can feel as if we are one.'

But before getting involved with someone else, the first step to intimacy was to be intimate with ourselves, Jan explained.

'Intimacy starts with listening, getting to know and accept ourselves, and learning how to be with ourselves. Then we can start to reveal our inner world to another person and to show them who we are and see them as they are. Nothing is hidden.'

To help us get in touch with our inner worlds, Jan employed the assistance of some strawberries.

The strawberries were passed around while Jan told us that beetroots were also available for those with strawberry allergies. Then the plinky plonky music came back on.

'Breathe, stay connected to yourself and really look at the strawberry,' Jan was saying. 'Look at it as if you've never seen a strawberry before. See every detail.'

I examined the seeds of the strawberry and thought that they looked like whiteheads. I thought about how satisfying they would be to squeeze out.

'Bring it closer and smell it,' said Jan.

I brought it to my nose and remembered a toy I had as a kid called Strawberry Shortcake. I pulled it away to look more closely at it and it began to look cartoon-like, with its technicolour red and dents and shine and —

'Bring the strawberry to your lips and feel the sensation of it touching lightly, feeling the coolness of the strawberry and its texture on your lips. Stay open to the feelings and sensations that arise,' said Jan.

I brought the strawberry to my lips, and its firm and plump flesh felt sexy – but then my mind kicked in: *You can't find a strawberry sexy! Pull yourself together! Stop feeling turned on by a strawberry!*

'Very gently rub the strawberry against your teeth so that the smallest drop of juice is released. Let the taste of it fill you. Then, allow a tiny piece of the flesh of the strawberry into your mouth. Keep tasting, smelling, seeing, feeling, breathing. Take as long as you can to stay present with the experience of the strawberry,' said Jan.

I put the strawberry against my teeth and tasted the juice, but would not allow myself to get lost in this strawberry orgy.

Jan invited us to notice all our thoughts and feelings about the strawberry. She explained: 'This is your first intimacy – being aware of what is happening for you, how you feel, how you are breathing, your physical and emotional world. Being with ourselves and our body and all that is in it. You should never lose touch with this intimacy with yourself, even when you are with other people.'

As we snogged our strawberries, she explained that many of us found it hard to be with our own inner experience. Shock and trauma might mean that we have cut off from feelings and sensations. We turn the volume down on feelings of sadness and pain and anger if they feel too much for us, or for other people too.

'We settle for feeling a little less alive so that we are comfortable and fit in.'

These tantra workshops were a place where we could not just get in touch with others, but get in touch with ourselves.

I took a long, slow deep breath.

What feelings was I avoiding? Shame around feeling pleasure? Shame about being turned on, both with a strawberry and without? Shame at having to be the person who has to pay to learn how to do intimacy with a strawberry? Just shame full stop?

Those thoughts were uncomfortable, so I distracted myself by wondering if anyone in the room had made love to the beetroot instead.

The next part of the workshop involved being intimate with others. I caught eyes with my husband across the circle and then looked away and asked the man next to me if he wanted to work together.

These 'intimacy dates' lasted between fifteen minutes and two hours, and the structure was very simple. We were to sit with our partners and start each sentence with the words, 'I am aware . . .' and then say out loud something we were aware of from our outer world (what was in the room), our inner world (our bodily sensations) and our mental and emotional world. We were to take turns to share with total honesty our feelings in each moment. This, Jan explained, was what intimacy was. Total transparency with another human being.

I went into my full singing-and-dancing joke routine. Look how charming I am! I am not at all uncomfortable! No siree! Not me! I have just married a stranger who can't look at me, which is causing feelings in me I don't understand but let's just keep the show on the road!

'Notice the ways that you block intimacy,' Jan said, after that session. 'Did you make a joke?'

Yes.

'Did you make small talk – saying things that you've said before?'

Yes.

'Did you allow silences?'

No.

'Did you let the words that were spoken touch you?'

No.

'Did you try to please?'

Of course.

'Could you allow the feeling of not knowing what was going to come next? And the sometimes awkward feeling that can accompany that?'

No. I wanted to keep the conversations on track. Be in control.

It turned out that while I'd thought we'd had a great chat, none of this was actually intimacy.

Jan told us about the different stages of intimacy, as she saw it. The first stage involved losing our 'autopilot' conversation. We all have routines, she explained, when we meet someone new. Routines of the funny stuff we say, the clever stuff, the 'nice' stuff – all the conversational habits that we hope will make a good impression. These habits are not intimacy.

Likewise, we have routines with people we know and love. We have areas we don't talk about and areas we do. We get into certain patterns. Talking about the kids, the house, what we're watching on television. All these things are autopilot conversations.

Being intimate, she explained, meant you don't say all the stuff you normally say, you don't use your favourite jokes and well-worn stories, you don't slip into small talk or banter. You say honestly what is happening in that moment. It meant not trying to hide anything – including our fears or insecurities. It meant showing when something the other person said had impacted us or hurt us, or touched us. In other words, it was about dropping the need to be safe, cool and right. It meant dropping our armour.

It sounded awful.

The second stage of intimacy was to be willing to 'step into the unknown' with this person, to let go of controlling the interaction and let something unexpected unfold. We were invited to allow silences, because out of the silences comes real communication and connection.

Finally, we had to take all of this very slowly.

She explained that we lived in a fast-paced society, so we are habituated to doing everything fast and intensely. This can be useful in life, but in our relationships it meant that we were not really connecting or communicating with each other. Only by slowing down could we feel calm and grounded enough to really meet the other person . . . and to meet life. I had failed on every count.

The next day, I partnered up with a woman with long hair and a willowy yoga body. We sat opposite each other on cushions and crossed our legs. She had a steady gaze and it made me squirm. This time I was aware of everything I did to block intimacy, but I seemed powerless to stop it.

'I am aware of your eyes,' she said. 'They are very blue.'

'I am aware of your eyes too,' I said quickly, to avoid any awkward silences.

'I am aware of feeling a warmth in my stomach,' she said.

'I am aware that I like your top,' I said, again too quickly. *Fill the silence! Give her a compliment! Be nice!*

'I'm aware of wanting to sit closer to you,' she said.

I didn't want to sit closer. Why did she want to sit closer to me? What did she want from me? I instantly decided that she was clingy and needy and weird.

'Sure!' I smiled. 'We can do that!' My voice went higher as I lied. It was a highness I heard a lot. The highness of 'being nice'. The highness used every time I said 'Sure, whatever you want!', or 'Yeah! Whatever! I'm easy! No problem!'

'I'm aware that I am thinking you don't want that,' she said, totally calmly.

'I'm aware that I don't really but if you want to, it would be OK.' Now I started criticizing myself for making such a big deal of her wanting to sit closer. What's wrong with you, Marianne? Just give her what she wants. Don't be selfish. And what difference does it make if she sits closer?

Jan's voice reminded us to 'notice whether you are staying with yourself or whether you are fully focused on the other person. Can you stay with yourself *and* be with the other person?'

No, I could not. Staying with myself and being with another person was like trying to pat my head and rub my tummy at the same time. When I was with another person, I stopped existing – it was all about them. Were they OK? What did they want? What did they need? Was I accommodating that?

No wonder I wanted to run away.

'Notice if you have stopped breathing,' Jan said.

I had stopped breathing. Jan explained that shallow breathing is one of the ways we cut off from difficult feelings. It's our way of shutting down. How often did I do this around people?

'Take some deep, slow breaths,' Jan suggested.

I did, and with each breath I let go of some of the tension I was holding in my body.

'I notice I've been clenching my hands, and my jaw,' I said. 'And my shoulders feel stiff.'

She nodded, and it felt good to notice that and say it out loud.

'I'm aware of your hair,' she said. 'It's catching in the light.'

This time I forced myself to leave a pause and I took another deep breath to let the words 'land', as Jan would say.

'I'm aware of the wooden floor,' I said, still looking at it.

'I'm aware that I'd like to get to know you better. I want to be your friend.'

'I'm aware that that makes me feel stressed,' I said, looking at her. I felt like I was being electrocuted with her eyes.

I waited for her to get angry, but she didn't. She simply nodded.

It hit me then how much I thought that speaking any truth would make people angry and how terrified I was of that. I was always pleasing, placating, managing, trying to keep things 'nice'. Like a little girl, I was always waiting for someone to shout and get angry with me and I danced in circles to avoid it. It was exhausting.

'I'm aware that the room is warm and I feel heat in my chest,' she said, unaware of the turmoil this tiny interaction was causing in me.

'I'm aware that I feel like you want something from me that I cannot give,' I blurted out. Again, I waited for her to get upset with me, but she didn't. She simply heard me. It was a relief. Why wasn't she getting angry with me? It hit me that as well as fearing people's anger and disappointment, I was also always thinking that they wanted more from me than I had to give.

'I'm aware that I don't want anything from you but to connect at this moment,' she replied with a gentle smile on her face.

Oh.

Underneath the story I'd made up was a sadder story.

'I'm aware that I don't know why you would want to connect with me,' I said and felt the hot prick of tears, which I tried to push down by pinching my thumb with the nail of my index finger, a trick from childhood to stop me from getting upset. Why would anyone want me around if I wasn't doing things for them? Being nice? Pleasing?

'Notice when you cut off your energy, when your feelings are too strong,' Jan was saying into her mic. 'Strong feelings might feel like that lump in your throat, that feeling you get when you're at the top of a roller coaster.'

I hated roller coasters.

And I was cutting off my feelings – or at least trying to. If I could just focus on the pain of the nail digging into the flesh, I'd be OK, I'd be able to get out of this situation without crying . . . but why was it so important that I didn't cry in front of someone? Also, why was I always trying to 'get out' of situations – get away from people?

I was always trying to keep control, I saw. To pretend that things were not impacting me when they were. I didn't want to be weak and vulnerable in front of people. Weak and vulnerable people were annoying. Needy.

The bell went to signal the end of the session.

I went to the loo and cried on my own.

My next meeting was with a man who I knew from other retreats. He was a big talker, so I sat back and let him do the work – talking, talking, talking about all the things he was aware of. There was no need to worry about silence this time because he was filling it, so I just smiled and nodded. I congratulated myself on what a saint I was being by listening to him, while also judging him for being a selfish prick who just wanted to talk about himself.

'I am aware that you hide behind silence,' he told me. It felt like a punch in the guts.

My last meeting was with the man I'd found attractive at the first tantra retreat. The one whose hand I touched in the first exercise.

Panic meant that I did everything I was not meant to do.

I over-talked, allowed no silences, I brought out all my best witty, self-deprecating jokes. I couldn't shut up . . . until—

'I'm aware this conversation does not feel honest,' he said after about ten minutes.

'Oh.'

'I'm aware that I don't trust you,' he said.

'Oh.'

He told me that he got the vibe that I was attracted to him and he did not feel the same way back.

And at first it felt liberating actually – to just get this out in the open, all this subtext that goes on between people – do you fancy me, do you not? Do I fancy you, do I not? Here it was, just out there. He wasn't into me. So what?

But it kept coming.

'I feel like you come at me with . . .' he did this motion with his arms, which looked like a bear on the attack.

'Oh.'

'You have a very strong energy.'

'Oh.'

'I'm aware that I experience you as having a very strong energy,' he corrected himself.

I wanted this to stop.

'I'm aware that I am not happy,' he said.

'I'm aware that I'm not happy either,' I replied.

'I'm aware that feels like the first honest thing you've said.'

The next morning I woke up with puffy eyes from crying. I felt like I'd been skinned alive. My silent, listening saint role busted. My over-talking, clever, funny role a sham. My fear of rejection from a hot man made real. Again.

I wanted to run away.

My husband had come up to me after the evening sessions

asking if I needed a hug or a cup of tea, but I felt too embarrassed for him to see me so upset. I told him I was fine and just needed to go to bed. At breakfast I had pretended not to see him and sat outside on my own with a bowl of muesli.

We sat as a group in a big circle as Jan explained why intimacy could be so painful – it is a risk to really show yourself to another person. In that moment we become vulnerable, unprotected, open to being hurt, and open to all the fears and demands of another. They could walk away, reject us, ridicule us, or they could want more than we had to give. They could engulf us, so that we lose ourselves in them and forget we have a separate existence.

'So of course we are scared of intimacy. But in avoiding it and protecting ourselves, we also prevent ourselves from ever being really seen and loved,' Jan explained.

I started crying when she said this. It was like two taps had been turned on. I kept crying as she explained that the trick was not to try to banish the fear of intimacy, but to welcome it as *part* of intimacy.

'Give your fear a soft, welcoming place and embrace it,' Jan said. Allow yourself to be scared. Speak it to the other person. We need to trust the other person, but mostly we need to trust in ourselves, to trust that even if we get hurt, we will be OK. 'Intimacy is about trusting that our hearts are bigger than our wounds,' she said. 'It's scary . . . but worth it.'

Over the next week we would be given a crash course in the dynamics of how humans relate to each other. I wished that someone had taught us this stuff at school. It would have saved so much pain and been infinitely more useful than quadratic equations.

We were taught about 'triggers' – or why certain people pissed us off.

Jan explained that the people who trigger you often show some behaviour that you don't like in yourself – or that you don't allow in yourself. So if someone was really loud and chatty and it drove you crazy, it could be that you were also loud and chatty and felt bad about it, or it could be the opposite – that you didn't allow yourself to speak up and were jealous of their loudness and chattiness.

'Yes, but can't someone just be annoying?' someone asked. Sometimes, yes, but generally, no. Someone who drives one person crazy won't bother another person at all, and vice versa. Their behaviour is the same; our reactions are very different.

We were then invited to think about someone who annoyed us in the room. One immediately came to mind: there was a woman who really irritated me; she seemed so vulnerable, so needy . . . I wanted to come out of my skin just being near her. I wanted to tell her to pull herself together. Toughen up, woman!

We were then invited to do the unimaginable. We could go up to the people who annoyed us and tell them why. We were to position it in a way that made it clear the problem was with us, not them.

There was no way I was going to do that. No way.

But just as I was about to leave the room to hide in the loo, the weak, annoying, vulnerable, needy woman seemed to be walking my way. She sat opposite me, plopping down onto a cushion.

'Um,' she said, looking at me with big, watery eyes. 'Um. I find you quite hard to be around . . . Because, I suppose I see a lot of vulnerability in you and I find that hard. I find you to be quite . . . um . . . needy, I suppose.'

What the hell was she talking about? I wasn't vulnerable! Or needy! I'd spent my whole life trying not to be needy! My sister said I despised needy people! Miss Independent, that was me!

She was wrong! I was nothing like her. *At all.*

Except, of course, I was.

I was needy. I needed people to like me. I needed them to approve of me. I needed to be wanted and considered 'good'. I needed men to fancy me so that I felt attractive.

I went back to the dorm and sat on my bed. I thought about the hot guy who'd told me that he didn't trust me. He triggered me because he was hot and made me feel . . . well, not hot. When I was near him, I felt like an awkward teenager that nobody wants to dance with. A sweaty ginger minger.

Did I just need to make peace with the teenage part of me that feels ugly and wrong? Or own my hotness around him?

One of my roommates came in and sat down on her bed.

'So basically . . . what's she's saying with this triggering stuff is that I'm the dickhead,' she said. 'I always think it's them, but it's me.'

'Yeah, I think so.'

For the rest of the day that line stayed in my head.

I'm the dickhead.

That evening, after a dinner of yet more mushrooms, we were invited to share how we were feeling in groups of four. My husband was in the group. Well, my ex. We had passed our twenty-four-hour mark, and when Jan had declared that the marriages were now dissolved, I looked around and couldn't see him anywhere.

When it came to my turn to speak, I started crying. 'I hate it here. I want to run away . . . I feel trapped.'

They listened with kind faces.

'Why do I find this so hard? Why can't I just be with people? I'm always terrified someone is going to tell me something I don't want to hear, something that hurts me. I always think people want more of me than I have to give – but maybe that's not even true, it's just in my head. I'm scared of you all, that's the truth. I'm always waiting for you to attack me. Which I know is stupid, but it's how I feel.'

'What would it take for you to trust and to open your heart?' my ex-husband asked.

'I need to go slow and feel safe,' I found myself saying. Which surprised me. I never did anything slowly. I could see that in the past year I'd done what I always did – I'd flung myself into loads of new experiences, often experiences that were too much for me to handle. Throwing myself in at the deep end was a protection mechanism – it meant that I didn't have to feel anything, I could get lost in intensity, rather than experiencing the tender, awkward joy of intimacy. I had done this all my life.

'Would you like a hug?' he asked.

I did.

In his arms, I felt so tired. Tired of the self I've been – the singular self that was always 'on' with others, always on red alert for conflict, always trying to make things OK and braced to run away as soon as they weren't.

My body softened and I sighed. I cried and cried and cried . . . I'd never let go in front of a man like this, never been held like this before.

'I'm sorry I ran away from you,' I said.

'I ran away too,' he replied.

'Would you like to do an intimacy meeting together? I have a private room, we could do it there,' the ex said. I noticed for the first time how beautiful his face was, how blue his eyes were.

I said yes and followed him through the grounds into a wing of buildings I hadn't been to before. We walked into his very tidy room.

'Is this OK?' he asked.

'It's OK with me – is it OK with you?'

'Yes, it's nice. Do you want to sit on the bed? Maybe we could face each other – would that work?'

'Yes, OK.'

We sat on the bed, both cross-legged, a few inches apart.

We breathed again and looked at each other. We were now so close I could feel his breath. I could see how normal me would have overpowered this gentle man. Gone into a whole song-and-dance routine. But now there was no power left in me.

There was no pretending. No impressing. No defending.

Just me and him in his room.

He seemed nervous, and a part of me was irritated. I wanted him to be strong and in control. And then I remembered what Jan had said about how what irritates you in another is usually something you don't like or suppress in yourself. I was nervous too, and trying not to be.

'Shall we start?' he said.

'Yes,' I said.

'Would you like to start?'

'OK.' I took a deep breath. 'I'm aware of the light . . .' I looked at the bedside light.

'Shall we turn the light off?'

'No,' I said automatically. Don't make a fuss, don't change anything, I'm easy . . . but then I realized that the light was bothering me. 'Actually, do you mind if we do?' I said, worried that this request made me fussy and pathetic.

'Of course,' he said.

He turned it off.

'I'm aware that feels better,' he said.

I nodded and looked into his ocean eyes.

'I'm aware of your long eyelashes,' I said.

He nodded as he took that in.

'I'm aware I'd like to look at you,' he said. 'Is that OK?'

Nobody had asked me that before. *Can I look at you?* It seemed like such an important thing to do, to ask in this way.

'Yes,' and as soon as I said 'yes', the fear kicked in that he would not like what he was looking at.

'I'm worried I don't look good enough,' I said.

He nodded as if to say he heard me, not that he agreed with me.

'I like looking at you,' he said. Again, the simplicity of his words touched me. *I like looking at you.*

He kept looking, but it was a soft look. He was not drilling holes into my eyes. He was not playing intimacy mind-games.

'I'm aware of your blue eyes,' he replied.

My heart pounded with the attention.

'I'm aware my heart is pounding,' I said.

'I'm aware that my heart is racing,' he replied.

'I'm aware that I don't know what to say,' I said.

For a few seconds we sat in silence.

'I'm aware I'd like to stroke your arms,' he said.

It didn't sound like a demand, or even a request. Just a desire. I felt no pressure to oblige but I wanted him to touch me.

'Yes,' I said. 'Sorry, I'm aware I'd like that.'

He stroked my arms, so slowly and gently. I shivered and closed my eyes.

How could this tiny gesture feel so immense?

Then a voice kicked in – *this isn't enough for him, he wants to do something more, you have to give him more! You are boring him! He doesn't want to sit here stroking your arms! He is just being nice! You should do something more interesting!*

'I'm aware that I'm thinking you don't want to be here and this is boring for you.'

'I'm aware that I want to be here.'

'OK,' I said, but I worried he was just being nice.

'I'm worried you are just being nice,' I said.

'I'm not.'

'OK.'

'I'm aware I'd like to keep stroking your arm.'

'OK.'

And it was so beautiful, this stroking of my arm. It was exquisite, but the voice in my head wanted to fight it: *What is he getting out of this? How can he possibly enjoy this? You are doing nothing for him. Do something, Marianne!*

'Breathe,' he whispered. And usually, if someone told me to breathe I wanted to punch them, but this time I didn't.

I breathed.

'I'm aware I'd like to stroke your neck,' he said.

'Yes.'

As his fingers brushed my neck, I moaned. Never had anything in my life felt so tender.

I didn't deserve to be touched like this.

He kept looking at me.

'I don't understand why you want to be here with me,' I said.

A tear rolled down my cheek and he reached over to my face and wiped it away. He kept looking at me.

'I don't know what to do,' I cried.

'You don't have to do anything.'

I felt so young and stupid and powerless.

'I'm scared,' I said. I closed my eyes. I felt scared that I was not enough for him, that I felt out of control, that . . . that I was an inept, sexually inadequate girl who was out of her depth. I realized how much this fear was with me still, even after all the workshops – a deep fear of not being good enough. Of not knowing what to do.

'Stay with me, open your eyes . . .' he said. The slight, geeky man from the workshop had vanished and in his place was a steady, strong force who knew exactly what to do.

He moved his hand so that it sat on my heart.

'Stay with me. Breathe. Look at me.'

I looked into his blue eyes, which seemed to contain a whole world.

'Stay with me, breathe,' he said.

I breathed. And breathed. And breathed. I kept looking into his eyes.

'I'd like to stroke your arms,' I said.

I got lost in stroking the outline of his arms. It was like tracing my finger over a new landscape, a desert. The light tan of his skin and the pale underside, the soft hairs . . . each touch felt like entering another world, and at the same time, it felt like home.

What an honour it was, to touch someone. How beautiful skin was.

I kept touching him and breathing. He kept touching me and breathing. We were breathing together. At some point I stopped being me and he stopped being him and I had the vision that we were entwined like the yin and yang symbol, flying through the night sky . . . And it felt like we were completely equal, there was no power play. Normally with men I had this feeling of being inferior or superior – there was a power game going on. This was so completely different – we were equal. We were one.

When I got up, it felt like my feet were not on solid ground. It was like when you get off a rocky boat and find yourself in a new country.

We spent the rest of the week listening to each other as a group. Really listening. Listening not to respond or to give advice or to fix, but listening simply to experience what it was like to be in that other person's world.

We would then repeat back what we'd heard and they would say 'yes', or correct us if what they had said was different to what we had heard, which was often the case.

People blossomed as they spoke and we listened. Some said things they'd never said before. The words could come because they knew they would be met with love and acceptance. I thought of my experience of this at the woman's circle, the radical power of simply being listened to, of being heard and seen.

I realized that listening to each other, really listening, was a huge act of love. Setting aside our own thoughts, beliefs and agendas long enough to really listen to another, to be physically, emotionally and mentally present with another, had near-magic effects. Allowing the fact that this person had their own world, their own experience, that was different to ours. Allowing ourselves to listen without judging or comparing. Allowing ourselves to listen in a way that allowed us to be changed by what we heard.

How often we speak and listen and miss each other completely, each lost in their own world of people-pleasing and defensiveness.

I learned that the concept of 'people-pleasing' is a learned behaviour that starts in childhood. Growing up, we have two needs: for authenticity and connection. So we need to be ourselves, and we need love. If by being ourselves – by crying, moaning, clinging – we feel like love is cut off from us, we will always choose connection over authenticity. And so a life of denying our real feelings begins. It becomes so second-nature we might not even know we are doing it. But pleasing people is a way of avoiding intimacy, because you are never showing people the real you.

Here, we were encouraged to keep being honest with others about what was going on within us. In between exercises we were invited to talk to the individuals we might have had problems with. 'If your heart is closed to one person, it's very likely to be closed to everybody,' Jan said. 'Often, once we air the problem, it dissolves.' This terrified me, but the difference it made was vast.

'It hurt me when you didn't open the door for me this morning,' I found myself ashamed to admit to somebody. 'It made me feel like I was invisible.' They would look on with kind eyes and the grudge would disappear, along with all the stories I'd been building around it.

We were encouraged to regularly check in on how we were feeling. Did we really want to be doing what we were doing? Were we going into people-pleasing mode? Did we need space? Did we need a hug? Did we need quiet? Were we then able to ask for those things? To look after ourselves?

I could see that for so long, I had made myself feel wrong for having needs – particularly my need for space – and so I had flipped between losing myself in people, doing everything I thought they wanted me to do, and running a mile in a state of resentful exhaustion.

When I looked after myself, being with others did not

become the strain it often was otherwise. In fact, it was a joy. A soft place to land.

On the last evening, Hawaiian Santa, in his hot-orange shirt, sang to us: *'The greatest gift you'll ever learn is just to love and be loved in return.'* As we all listened, lying on the floor like children in playschool, I looked around the room.

A man was crying into another man's arms.

A couple were sitting next to each other, holding hands. They had had a hard week, saying things to each other that they had been keeping back for years. The woman had announced that she was pain-free for the first time in eight years of suffering from a chronic health problem.

'I think that everything I was keeping in was making me sick,' she said, shocked by the power of this revelation. She, like me, was a people-pleaser, a bottle-upper. 'There was violence in my silence,' she admitted. 'It was hurting him and hurting me.'

The oldest man in the group, a man in his late seventies, had the shining face of a young boy. Everyone looked different.

I didn't realize how much we wore our pain on our faces – rictus grins pretending everything was OK, scowls to keep people away – and in our bodies . . . how rigidly we usually hold ourselves, braced for impact, prepared for anything, so that nothing could hurt us as it did when we were defenceless children who walked into the world with open eyes and soft bodies and trusting the world, until the day something – a teacher's shout, a parent's absence – made us feel the danger of the world.

'Don't trust people,' was the advice my dad gave his three daughters. With good reason – he had been hurt time and time again and he wanted to spare us that. 'Never rely on people,' said our mother, also trying to protect us from the financial dependence she and many of her generation had

had to have on men. Throughout the workshop I had heard people talk about being hurt in ways that I had not been hurt. I was grateful for the protection I had, unwittingly, built around me. But it was time to let some of that protection down. I had missed out on too much of life because of it.

I looked around again.

People's faces relaxed and lit up, their bodies unfurled, they looked sparkly and alive and conversation flowed between people who, in the normal world, would not know how to connect. Our true selves were shining, and it was beautiful. Everyone was beautiful. I loved them all. It was impossible not to love people's true essence. This was what was real, I thought.

Any damage done in a relationship needs to be healed in a relationship, Jan had said. This week we had been healing each other.

When it came to my turn to speak in the final circle, I felt the eyes of everyone gaze on me.

'I'm tired of being me. I'm ready to be part of a "we".'

14

We Made Love

I arrived at Paddington Station in a state of love. I walked past confused tourists and stressed-out commuters, pulling my wheelie bag and smiling at everyone. No one smiled back.

The difference between the 'real' world and Jan's world was stark.

I remembered something I'd read about the opposite of love not being hate but fear. That's what I saw on people's faces: fear. Heads down, eyes locked on screens, ears covered with headphones. Bodies bowed like modern-day Lowry figures.

I stopped and ordered a coffee at Costa. The young guy behind the till didn't look at me as he took my order. Normally I wouldn't even have noticed this. Today it cut like a knife.

I once read a study that found that every time somebody blanks us in public – even someone we don't know – it makes us feel disconnected, and this disconnection is linked to depression, high blood pressure and dementia. In cities this was happening to us all day, every day.

Real life hurt.

On one table next to me, a young woman wearing giant pink headphones was looking at her laptop, which was playing a TV show I didn't recognize. She was hermetically sealed into her own little world. Suddenly, I was in tears in the coffee shop at how much we'd fucked things up. We humans in this modern world. No wonder we were so lonely, so lost.

I looked out at the concourse at smartly dressed men and women, marching with great purpose, anyone who stood in their way or walked too slowly an obstacle to be scowled at. I thought about people accessing dating apps in this hurried, stressed, fearful state. It struck me that to truly connect with each other, the way we had in the workshop, we needed time and tenderness, so completely at odds with the modern world.

But then, hope. A mother was stroking her child's glossy hair as she gazed up at train times. An older woman was squeezing a young man with a big rucksack and giving him a kiss on each cheek before letting him walk away into the crowd, off on an adventure.

Small moments of love sprouting from the concrete.

It was always an adjustment, coming from a retreat or festival back into the city. What we did in the workshops was so far from normal life, and yet it felt much more real than the way most of us were living. I struggled to know how to bring the feelings I had had in tantra, and the way of relating to people I had learned, into my day-to-day life. I kept thinking of the words I'd spoken on the last day. 'I want to be part of a "we".'

What did that mean?

Did that mean a couple or that I just wanted to be less cut off from others?

Over the next few weeks, my ex-twenty-four-hour-husband, whose name was George, and I texted. He was planning to be in London for a work thing and wondered if he could stay for a few nights afterwards. 'On the sofa, no expectations?'

I promptly went into a tailspin of excitement and fear. Then the avoidant stuff kicked in. I spent the day before he arrived cleaning the bathroom, listing all the reasons he was not boyfriend material: he was skinnier than me, vegan, spiritual, used phrases like 'my inner boy' and 'sexy man' – and he didn't drink.

Then, while hoovering, I flipped to all the reasons I was not good enough for him: I wasn't pretty or skinny enough for him, and I was a horrible, evil meat-eater, who also consumed coffee, sugar and booze . . . and bought single-use plastic and got on planes and led a generally selfish life.

Attached had told me that all this overthinking and fault-finding was a sign of my avoidance. My job was now to focus on his good qualities instead of finding reasons to reject him. And there were many good qualities . . . he was clever and kind, and campaigned to save the world.

I remembered a piece of advice Jan had given one of the group: Don't shut yourself down until you meet the right guy, because you don't know when that's going to be. In the meantime, keep your heart open to people. Lean in to pleasure. Take lovers, go on dates, meet different people, keep your heart open . . . but always go slowly enough that any hurt you experience is not insurmountable. Don't jump in. Take your time. Lean on your girlfriends. Put your first intimacy first – always.

What I found tricky about romantic and sexual relationships was this pressure to define what they were so early on. With friendships you could just hang out and it would develop any old way. But with romantic stuff the whole '*What is this?*' stuff hung in the air and messed with my head.

Jan distinguished between lovers and someone you were having a relationship with. Lovers could be loving, and you could have 'heart-centred' sex with them, but you were not building a life together, and you could have more than one at a time. Relationships meant that you were working towards a future together.

I hoped George could be a lover, but I felt shy about using the word. As I thought about all this, I scrubbed every inch of the flat. Whatever happened between us, at least having a lover made me mop my floors.

I called Rachel to tell her about my guest.

'Is he legal?'

'What do you mean?'

'How old is he?'

'My age.'

'OK, good.'

'Why did you ask that?'

'After your art guy.'

'Oh yeah. No, he's a grown-up – but he's a Buddhist.'

'Do Buddhists have orgasms?'

'Yes, but they don't kill mosquitos.'

'Right.'

I spent the days before George's arrival reading and underlining a book a tantra friend had given me, called *The Heart of Tantric Sex* by Diana Richardson. Inside, she had inscribed the message: *Here's to beautiful sex!* – something I'd said I yearned for.

The book, like many others, had been left at the bottom of my bed, unread. But now I had a man on his way and I was going to have beautiful sex! Maybe. Or maybe not. Maybe he really would want to stay on the sofa or the blow-up bed I'd bought on Amazon which slowly deflated throughout the night. I hoped he wouldn't want to do that.

The book promised 'a completely new way of making love', in which sex was something you sank into rather than did. It talked about scrapping goal-oriented, orgasm-chasing sex, based on friction and excitement – and instead, prioritized floating into a slow, gentle connection through deep breathing, eye-gazing and long hugs. It sounded like sexual nirvana.

My period arrived the day before he did.

Then a mouse.

He was wearing outdoor walking trousers, the kind with pockets, and a North Face waterproof. He looked like the kind of guy who would know which way north was in an apocalypse.

'Your hair is different,' he said.

'Oh yeah, I got it done.'

I'd had my roots done and the colour was a bit more mahogany than usual and it had been blow dried. I had got my blackheads squeezed and removed my chin hair in good light and plucked out one random long hair from my neck. I hadn't removed my leg hair properly. I was going to leave it, on account of being a liberated woman no longer dominated by the patriarchy, but then I lost my nerve and did a half-shave in the shower with a blunt razor and now I had a rash.

I wanted him to tell me I looked nice but he didn't.

I worried that he'd think I was fat and ugly in the real world, and I was aware that I was a good inch taller than him and infinitely broader than him. He had the lean body of a dancer or a rock climber. I had the body of a comfortable sofa. But he knew this, didn't he? He'd seen me before.

I was so self-conscious I found it hard to look him in the eye. I noticed that I always found this bit tricky – the 'hello' bit. And the goodbye bit, for that matter. Transitions are hard, he had said when we said goodbye at the end of the workshop.

I showed him up the dirty stairs, past Michael's 'Gone Fishing' sign and a notice outside the new downstairs neighbour's flat that announced 'Women Don't Owe You Shit'. I still hadn't met them.

I opened the door to my flat and felt surprised to see it so tidy. I'd been to the pound shop and bought a lot of candles, which were now scattered about the place. My sister was worried that I was going to set the place on fire.

He put down his rucksack and started looking at the books on my shelf. I offered him tea. We made small talk. Or rather, in my case, quick talk. My nerves were getting to me and I couldn't slow down. I was doing my one-woman comedy act, fake laughs, no silences, autopilot central.

This was not intimacy.

'Do you want to take a few breaths together?' he asked.

I felt embarrassed that it was obvious I was so nervous, and also relieved that he was staging a gentle intervention. I sat on the sofa next to him and we took a few deep, slow breaths together. It helped. It was actually amazing how much it helped.

'You OK?' George said.

'Yes,' I lied.

'I'm going to ask the dreaded question,' he said.

I racked my mind for what the dreaded question was.

'OK.'

'What's on your mind?'

I spat it out: 'I have a mouse and my period.'

'OK.'

'It appeared this morning when I was cleaning up. It just darted in front of the sofa and I went to the pound shop and got one of those humane traps but it hasn't run into it yet so it must still be running around the flat. So I'm sorry if a mouse appears.'

He shrugged. 'I think they're everywhere in London, aren't they?'

'I don't know. Yeah, maybe.'

Silence.

'And how do you feel about period sex?' I asked.

'That it's sex during a period? What do you mean?'

'Is it a problem?'

'Not if it isn't for you.'

'OK.'

'I'm not saying we have to have sex, but it's just on my mind.'

He smiled. 'Thank you for telling me.'

We started kissing on the sofa, and at first I felt nervous and fat but soon I relaxed into it. With him there was no rushing from one base to another. Kissing was its own destination.

'I love this bit,' he said.

'Which bit?

'This bit above your lips,' he said, moving a finger to that little ridge between my nose and lips.

'I love your skin,' I said, stroking his forearms. 'It's so smooth.'

'Thank you.'

'How do you get it so smooth?'

'I eat a lot of avocados.'

'How many?'

'One a day.'

'That's a lot.'

'I love your bum too,' he said, reaching for it. 'It's the size of infinity . . . you have an infinite butt. It shakes.' He started shaking the bum encased by my too-tight jeans. 'It's like jelly.'

I wanted to tell him that he probably shouldn't comment on women's infinite butts but when he said it he really did make it seem like a compliment, so maybe he did like it. Did

men like infinite butts? If so, I wished I'd known that sooner –
it might have saved me a lot of bother.

After kissing and talking about the size of my bum, we
walked and went for dinner in a local Thai restaurant. He
talked about his charity work, and my mind opened up with
tales from his different world.

'You've got to get involved, haven't you?'

I nodded. I never got involved.

We walked home holding hands. I usually hated to hold
hands – it made me feel like I was in primary school – but
this time I liked it.

'You're welcome to stay on the sofa, or a blow-up bed, if
you don't want to share a bed,' I offered, hoping he didn't
want this.

'I'd like to sleep with you, if that's OK,' he said.

'Yes, it's OK, I was just checking.' I was relieved and now
nervous.

Alas, it turned out he really did just want to sleep. He
unpacked his own pillow (he had allergies and a bad neck)
and his own sheet (duvets were too heavy for him) and went
out like a light.

I lay awake wondering what I'd done wrong.

When I woke up in the morning, he had turned away
from me.

His body was a closed door.

We had some half-hearted kissing but there was no fire
between us. I wanted it to be all yin-yang ecstasy and flying
over deserts, but the spell was broken.

We tried to have sex but it didn't work.

'Sex never really gives you what you think it's going to give
you,' he said. 'What is penetration, anyway?'

He was right.

Penetration had never given me what I thought it would give me. It took me until my forties to learn that while penetrative sex helps men to orgasm and women to get pregnant, it does not usually lead to a good time for women. In fact, seventy per cent of women cannot orgasm through penetration alone. Nobody had told me this. I thought that there was something wrong with me for not enjoying some of the sex I'd had. But still, I did the sex I thought I was meant to do to make men happy. If they were happy, I was happy.

And so I felt disappointed that we had not gone through with disappointing sex. Why? Because I wanted him to want me. Even if I didn't enjoy the sex, I wanted him to enjoy it.

Instead he offered to make breakfast.

'I'm sorry if I disappointed you,' he said, over breakfast.

'You didn't,' I lied, a fake smile on my face.

'Are you sure?'

'Yes, I'm sure!' I lied again.

'OK,' he said, unconvinced.

I didn't know what to say next – we were in a conversational dead-end, after he'd been brave enough to say the truth and I was meeting it with a fake smile. Why did I do this? Why did I go so silent with men? With everyone? Enough, Marianne, enough.

'Well, I was a bit disappointed. I'm worried it's because now that you're here you don't find me attractive.'

He nodded. 'Would you like a reality check?' he asked, using a phrase that Jan had told us to use when our heads were imagining all sorts of things. Ask the other person for a reality check, she'd suggested.

'Yes.'

'I find you attractive and I like you – it's just that sometimes

I get stressed and my body, well – it doesn't do the things I want it to do.'

I nodded. Men had talked in the workshops about the pressure they felt to perform and the shame they felt in not being able to.

Jan said that any time we started an intimate relationship, fears would come up. Fears about the person, and fears about performance and expectations. Fears based on relationships gone by. She said it was helpful to voice them all.

'Shall we just say everything that's on our minds?' I asked. 'Just get it out?' I could not believe I was the one suggesting this.

'Do you want to go first?'

'OK.' My tummy lurched. Jan had described intimacy as sometimes feeling like you were at the top of a roller coaster. That was how I felt now.

'Um, OK. I've been single most of my life, and so I don't feel like I'm very sexually experienced . . . and' – this made me want to puke – 'and I worry that I'm shit in bed and I'll be a disappointment.'

My cheeks were on fire. How had I just told a man I wanted to sleep with that I thought I was shit in bed? What kind of seduction technique was that?

He nodded and smiled.

'I, er . . . I sometimes find it hard to, er . . . perform.'

I nodded. 'The longest I've ever gone out with anyone is six months,' I said.

He nodded again, taking it in. 'Why is that, do you think?'

I hated this question. How many times had I been asked this question? Urgh.

'I dunno, I guess there were different things going on – I was probably quite scared of men, and sex, and also I never thought I was good-looking or the girl that guys liked . . . but

then also, when I did get in a relationship I felt trapped. So I
don't know. I like my freedom. I read this book that said that
I was a person who is "single at heart". I avoid relationships.'

'I'm anxious avoidant—'

'What does that mean again?'

'That I run away from relationships but also get clingy if I
feel someone moving away from me,' he said. I nodded and
wondered, not for the first time, if all this terminology was
helping or hindering us. Were we locking ourselves into these
labels?

'Sometimes I wonder if I'm capable of real love,' he added.

I'd never heard anyone say that before.

'I panic when people need me,' I said, repeating something
my sister had accused me of. Correctly.

'Me too,' he said.

'I'm afraid you're going to fall in love with me!' I found
myself saying, and then laughed at the ridiculousness of fearing that someone didn't fancy me and that they'd fall in love
with me at the same time.

'I'm afraid you're going to fall in love with me!' he said.

'OK, so let's not fall in love with each other,' I said.

'Deal.'

We kissed. It felt different to before. We were both really
there, no pretending or hiding, nothing to lose. Who knew
that confessing to what shit lovers we were would be so hot?

And so began five days – five days! – of the best sex of my
life. The beautiful, transcendent sex that I'd been dreaming
of. The stuff of poetry and art and gods, yin-yang signs and
stardust.

It was different to anything I'd experienced before, in that
a lot of it wasn't really 'sex' – or at least it wasn't penetration.

It was kissing and touching and eye-gazing, and it was so, so, so slow – it was like we'd entered some other time zone.

We lay and breathed and he stroked my body and I stroked his. We breathed some more. It was incredible how much the breathing made a difference. With each deep breath, I felt my body let go of things it didn't even know it was holding on to.

He touched me everywhere.

Long, slow, sweeping strokes on my arms and legs and tummy, and kisses everywhere. Stroking, nibbling, kissing – the neck, shoulders, waist, lips, ears, arms, thighs, inner thighs . . .

And as Jan had taught us to, I focused on my 'first intimacy'. I put all my focus on my own body, on feeling what was happening in it, rather than worrying about what was happening in his.

It was a whole new way of doing things. I thought my job in bed was to make sure the other person was having a good time, but this time I just focused on how I was feeling. It sounded selfish, but it worked. And I wasn't thinking of how my body was looking, only the sensations.

When he kissed my lips it was not so much a kiss as lips brushing together. It was slow and gentle. The kissing was a whole world of its own – wet and warm and deep. I got lost in his kisses. Our kisses.

One of the biggest revelations was how important breasts are. *The Heart of Tantric Sex* explains that they are the key to unlocking everything for women. They are our 'positive sexual pole' and they need to be awakened and stimulated in order to open up the rest of the body. For men it's the other way around – the positive sexual pole is the penis, which is why genital touch early on works better for men than women. On a woman if you go straight to the genitals it can feel like a smear test; it can take a long time to be ready for genital touch. How had it taken me till this age to know that?

He must have read this somewhere too, because he seemed to know it. He kissed my neck, my shoulders, my chest . . . before moving to my breasts, kissing them so gently. As he did, I felt currents of electricity move around my body.

In tantra retreats there had been a lot of talk of 'energy' and 'feeling energy moving', and most of the time I'd had no idea what they were talking about. It annoyed me, this 'energy' talk, it was so vague. But now I felt it – the more I breathed, I could feel different parts of my body tingle and then, sure enough, shots of energy would go up and down my body, like shivers. This must have been what was happening for Dr Quinn Medicine Woman.

He was going slower than I'd ever experienced. Hovering for what felt like hours with each kiss and touch. It was nothing like the sex I'd had before – the speedy box-ticking exercise that rushed to (his) orgasm.

And after that, things just started to happen.

Neither of us were 'doing' anything, but our bodies were moving anyway, of their own accord. A force was moving us.

I remembered Jan's advice that the more you breathe, the more you feel. So I kept breathing, deeply and slowly.

I didn't feel any need to perform and yet my body was doing things, compelled to touch him, kiss him, move in certain ways.

There were times when I thought I wanted penetration and then when he went to enter me, it was like my body said 'no'. I thought of all the times I'd overridden that feeling with men before. This time, I said I wasn't ready. I worried that he would run out of patience, but he didn't. Not at all.

We were honest.

'Does that feel good?' he asked as he stroked my hair.

'No,' I said.

We burst out laughing.

In the past, I would have started kissing and gone silent until the sex was over – but this time I didn't. We kept talking – 'Is my arm OK here?' 'Does that feel good?' 'I like the way you're kissing me there' – being able to say things out loud was a revelation. I was able to communicate. Tantra had given me a language to speak about things I'd had no idea how to speak about before.

Sex had so often been about performance, but this time it wasn't. We were getting things wrong, making mistakes – and that was what made it beautiful. Neither of us was trying to pretend to be something we weren't.

'I like that I don't feel like you're giving me all your moves,' I said at one point.

'That's because I don't have any moves,' he said.

'Me neither,' I said.

I told him about being shit at hand-jobs.

'It's the intention that matters, I think – how you feel when you're doing it,' he said.

I asked if I could practise on him.

He said I could and, while I moved to get into what I hoped would be a good position, I fell out of bed. I honestly fell out of the bed.

'You know what I'm going to ask . . .' he said.

'What?' I asked, from the floor.

'Did the earth move?'

I lay on the carpet giggling before getting up and trying again.

It felt like the first experience I never had and that I wished I'd had. We were both awkward and beautiful and innocent and hot.

And then at some point my body was craving him.

'Shall I get a condom?' he asked.

'Yes.'

He asked if I was ready for him to enter me. This was a thing in tantra – you must always ask a woman if she is ready. And in order to penetrate you must get not just a vocal yes, but a yes from her body. Women are often penetrated before we are ready, before we are open. I could not believe it had taken more than forty years to come across this concept – one that, surely, we should all be taught in school.

This time I was ready.

Once he was inside me I asked him to be still. We looked at each other.

According to *The Heart of Tantric Sex*, thrusting sex – the kind you see in porn and on TV – can be traumatizing. This pounding can be pleasurable when you're really turned on, but done too soon it's uncomfortable, painful and can lead to numbness. It can also cause a lack of sensitivity in men too. By being still, you give your body time to feel, and the chance to relax and become more sensitive. At first you might not feel much, but with time you will begin to regain feeling.

At first I worried the lack of motion would be boring for him, but the stillness made me feel close to him. We kept looking into each other's eyes. It felt like we were plugged in to each other.

The excitement came in shots – shots from the centre of my body, gentle fizzy shots, and they kept coming – like fireworks, but not strong and overpowering, just gentle explosions inside me.

There wasn't the whoosh of the usual orgasmic wave – nor the high of a clitoral orgasm – it was gentle and effortless and it kept coming . . . my body shook and shook and shook.

I felt self-conscious as he watched me, but his face was smiling, awed. Delighted. 'My electric lover,' he said.

And it kept coming, wave after wave after wave.

'That's how sex should be,' he said afterwards.

And it was. Finally, this was it. The sex I'd been dreaming of.

This sex was so far from the sex I'd seen on screen, where the man sticks it in and within a few seconds the woman is panting and moaning. Porn and mainstream films had made me think I should be wailing in pleasure after about ten seconds of thrusting. It was not so – never once had that happened to me, and for years I assumed the problem was mine. I thought that meant there was something wrong with me. There wasn't. The only thing wrong was the sex I'd been having.

Normal sex took place while drunk, and there was a formula – a bit of fingering, a blow job, him on top, me on top, a bit from behind, tick tick boom. And sometimes it was fine, sometimes it was nothing, sometimes it was sore. What it was not was beautiful.

I didn't blame men for the bad sex I'd had. Whenever they asked me what I liked, I didn't know the answer. And when something felt bad, I didn't tell them. I was putting on a performance. All I knew was what I'd seen in porn and on TV, where sex was something that was done *to* a woman, something fast and mechanical. And men were taking their cues from the same place. Of course, on an adult, rational level I knew that TV wasn't real, but on another level, I had absorbed those images. We all had. And so I'd put on a show, pretending I was having a great time, wanting him to come as quickly as possible so that we could stop and enjoy some hugs and kisses.

This sex was another thing entirely. This sex was touching and kissing and looking. It was not about coming, it was about connecting. It was not about doing, it was about relaxing. I realized that in tantra workshops I'd had utterly beautiful experiences while fully dressed – pleasure did not come from ticking sexual boxes. This sex wasn't about who was good or bad at what – it was about both of us being really there. Feeling everything. And I was feeling everything. The beauty of the streaky sky outside my window, the smoothness of his olive skin – it felt like everything had expanded. I was not lost in my head because I was saying everything out loud, no matter how messy or embarrassing the thoughts and fears were.

I remember Jan had once said that it was possible to make love to one inch of someone's arm and that you could bring someone to ecstasy by paying exquisite love and attention to someone's arm for hours. At the time I laughed at this idea. Now I understood.

What an honour it was to touch another body. What a privilege. And how easy it was, unwittingly, to hurt each other when we touched without tenderness or consciousness, thinking we were doing the things we were meant to do and missing each other in the process.

In some spiritual circles, sex was recognized as a path to the divine, and I could understand that now, too. The feeling of being one, of entering something that felt like a different dimension, well – it felt spiritual.

I thought of the nuns who had educated me and their vow of chastity, and the fear and shame that had been attached to this act of love.

What a shame. A huge, huge shame.

I didn't feel like I'd given something away with this sex, I felt like I was being filled up.

Now, if anyone asked me what I liked, I'd know the answer: I liked slow. Slow. Slow.

We went for hours, riding different waves.

'We're making love,' he said.

And we were. I'd never done that before. I'd had sex, but I'd never made love before.

He stayed for a week. He read me poetry and we slow danced. He cooked me vegan dinners and I bought him avocados and wrapped each one in a ribbon with a bow.

We had more beautiful sex.

George was an attentive and tender lover, but I realized that the difference was not just him – it was me, and how I felt in my body. All the breathing and workshops had made me sensitive in a way that I never had been before, so much so that a simple brush of his hand would make me shake.

We both marvelled at what was happening between us.

I'd read about the concept of accelerators and brakes when it came to sex. Accelerators are the things that turn us on, brakes are the things that turn us off. It's different for all of us. Some people might be turned on in nature while others want a darkened room. Some might get turned on by conversation, others by silence.

In our week together I learned a lot about what turned me on. Walks in the woods always did it – those sexy trees. Eating healthily made me feel happier in my body. Dancing together, music, movement made me feel in a state of flow. And feeling safe enough to say what I was feeling – this, I realized, was the biggest thing for me.

Because for all the bliss, there were painful moments too.

One day he asked if he could look at me, and as his eyes travelled around my body, looking like he was seeing something sacred, I started crying. 'I worry my body isn't good enough,' I said. He kept looking. 'I worry that I'm getting old.'

Another time I didn't want to have sex and I worried about saying no to him. Old conditioning kicked in that told me it was a woman's job to give a man what he wanted.

'I feel like I'm letting you down,' I said.

'Of course you're not. I don't want you to do anything you don't want to do. That wouldn't be good for me,' he said.

The sincerity with which he said those words broke something open in me. I started crying for all the women who were not able to say no, both in the past or now. I thought of what Daisy had said while I was reading *Pussy* – that there was collective trauma in women. Until the tantra workshops, I hadn't realized that I had always been scared of men. They were scary for their potential to reject, scary for the power they held everywhere, but also scary for their capacity to hurt me physically.

With George I felt safe. I had said difficult things and he never got angry with me. I didn't have to fawn or freeze. As I felt safer with him, I realized how unsafe I had felt with men before. The men I'd met over the past year had lessened my fear. I now saw us as brothers and sisters.

So much is held in our bodies.

You have a bad encounter with a sexual partner and your body remembers it.

But it felt like I was holding stuff in my body that wasn't even mine. It was the pain of the women who had come before me. It made no rational sense, but I gave myself up to all of it. I thought of another thing Jan had said: 'It is scary to meet with heart and sex.'

He kept holding me.

I kept saying what I was feeling.

But there was one thing I wasn't saying, even though the words wanted to jump out of my mouth every time I touched him. I worried that saying it would have to mean something, that it would be like signing a contract, or would mean that we had to be boyfriend and girlfriend, or that it would be something I regretted saying. But on our last night together, in bed, I blurted it out:

'I want to say something, but I don't want it to come attached to a whole story . . .'

'OK.'

'I love you.'

He paused and looked from me up to the ceiling.

'Thank you for saying that.'

15

Dumped

A couple of weeks later he told me that he wanted to step back. 'I want to take time to focus on my spiritual path,' he said.

'He actually said that?' said Rachel when I called her afterwards.

'Yeah, he said something about how he could feel me getting attached to him and that he felt conflicted because his ego liked the attention but he worried this relationship would take him away from his work.'

'What is his work?'

'Environmental stuff.'

'So what did you say?'

'I said "Fine, let's drop it", and pretended I didn't care.'

'Did you cry?' Rachel asked.

'No.'

'It's OK to be upset,' said Rachel. 'I'd be upset.'

'Yeah, I know,' I said.

I could cry over stuff on the telly. Cry at pretty much every self-help workshop I'd been to. But I couldn't cry over a man. Or maybe wouldn't. It was amazing how quickly the defence mechanism kicked in, this need to save face and not show that I'd been hurt. Even to myself.

My first reaction was to get back to work. I emailed every editor I knew pitching article ideas and sat at my computer for hours every day. I spurred myself on with a puritan fervour. I'd been wasting too much time with this love and sex stuff! I had been lazy! Bad! Wrong! It was time to get back to work. Stop wasting my time with men. Be a good girl.

Work did not let me down. Work made me feel like a good person.

At night, I went back to my usual bed companions: serial killer dramas and Instagram. Someone called 'Yonilicious' shared a cartoon of a woman wearing a T-shirt with the words: 'Masturbation never breaks your heart.'

For a moment I wondered if I should get back into the *Pussy* self-love and really feel all my feelings around the breakup. Do some swamping, rage and grieve with a bin bag.

I didn't do that. Instead, I did more work, watched more violent television and went to the pub, where I met an old journalism colleague in Soho and had five pints on an empty stomach.

'I'm getting a cold,' she said, as she plopped two vitamin C tablets into her beer.

It was a mark of how much my life had changed that getting naked with strangers now felt semi-normal, while going to a pub felt weird. I spewed the most unloving, unspiritual hate about George while I got Friday-night drunk.

It felt good.

Until it didn't.

The next day the tears and self-loathing came. All the old tapes went around in my head. Of course he couldn't love me. Why would he? That was for other people. Not me. I was too fat and ugly to be loved. Too loud. Too much.

Love was something that happened to other people. Not me. I went right back to the feelings I had after my doomed trip to Athens: that kind of love wasn't for me. It just wasn't.

As I sat on the loo, I itemized all my physical flaws and

vowed to address them. I would lose weight and sort out my hair. And maybe I'd get my teeth sorted. Finally get a brace and have them whitened. Then I'd pull someone new and really hot, and then George would see me out with him and regret his decision! That would show him!

For a few minutes I felt in control, and then it vanished. I wasn't in control. I might only have known George for a few weeks, but in that time I had done something I rarely do: I had opened my heart to him and he had said no, thanks.

It hurt. It made me feel sick. That kind of skinless, squirmy sick. And then I remembered a boyfriend I'd had in my twenties. My first boyfriend, really. I'd liked him a lot, and allowed myself to believe that maybe this was actually happening for me. Love. I remember calling Gemma and asking her how you know if you're in love. 'Do you think you are?' she'd asked. 'Yes,' I'd replied, shy and excited by this new reality.

A few days later he broke up with me.

I hadn't thought about that day in years. How skilled I seemed to be at blocking things out of my memory.

Was my whole life just a defence mechanism until this point? Did I actually want all the things that everyone else wanted? Quiet nights on the sofa, someone to hold hands with? Was the rest just an act? Had I just not allowed myself to want a partner because it was too painful to want something I didn't believe I deserved, or would ever get?

And then I started to cry, and for about four days I didn't stop. Something cracked. I wanted to make George the bad guy. Itemize every red flag he'd shown me. Make him the problem. But my pain wasn't about him – it was about disappointment and the fear I'd felt around men and love. Pain that I'd never allowed myself to feel because I was too busy pretending I was fine.

And then I remembered the moment that mum had

said she didn't think a husband and children were for me. I remember what my young teenage mind felt when she said it. I didn't hear that it wouldn't suit me – what I heard was that nobody would want me. I was not pretty in the way that my sisters and friends were, and no man would want to marry me.

I realized that I *was* just like everybody else. I wanted someone to talk to and to love and who loved me. I wanted someone to experience life with. Someone who would help me and I would help them. I was not special. I wanted to be loved and it made me feel weak to want it.

On Monday an envelope arrived with a book and a card with a drawing of a bunch of flowers on it. 'He was an idiot. I love you, as do so many others. Love, Rachel.' I teared up. I looked at the slim hardback book beneath the card. On the cover was a photo of the ocean, looking black and deep. Above the horizon, the name of the book: *Heartbreak*. It was a book by The School of Life, an organisation run by philosopher Alain de Botton that offered classes and published books aimed at giving people the emotional education they'd never had.

I would never have bought myself this book. I was too proud to admit that anyone could break my heart. I would not give them that power. I was better than that. Stronger than that.

Except, of course, I wasn't.

'Almost no one gets through life without having their heart broken,' the blurb read. 'Advice at such a dark moment tends to focus on letting time do the healing. But understanding and perspective also have a vital role.'

The opening chapter is called *Why Did They Leave Us?* and offers two reasons.

Number one: 'Despite what friends and well-meaning acquaintances tell us, we already know. It is us . . . They've gone because we weren't good enough.'

Exactly, Alain.

Number two: 'It is not that the relationship failed: we failed.'

Yes. Thank you for speaking the truth.

Of course, the book doesn't just blame us. It explains that we are all flawed when it comes to love. We hurt each other and ourselves, even when we have the best of intentions.

'Unfortunately for relationships, at least half the population is walking around with, and falling in love while beset by, a host of uncharted psychological issues that will make it hugely difficult for them to be predictable and well-attached in relationships.'

Oh. It continued:

'The ex may have been drawn to the warmth we offered them, but at the same time, our tenderness would have felt unfamiliar and been perceived as extremely threatening to parts of their personality. They may have struggled to understand what was going on inside themselves when they went cold and had to take their distance from us, but they lacked the tools . . . It may in the end have felt easier for them to blame us for being 'needy' rather than explore the complicated reasons why their own need was frightening to them . . .'

And then the book offered a consoling and tragic truth: 'They didn't manage to love us, but they probably couldn't, at this stage in their emotional evolution, love anyone that well, given the burden bequeathed by their unexplored past.'

I was so used to seeing my own problems, I had forgotten that other people have issues too.

I had had some of the most beautiful moments of my life with George, but there were also times when I looked into his eyes and I had the strong feeling that there was nothing there for me. But then I told myself that I was finding fault again; that this gut feeling wasn't really a gut feeling, it was my avoidance talking.

Why did I get drawn to these guys? Men who lived in other countries or who said from the off that they would not love me. Was my self-esteem so low? Was I so scared of something real I picked people who were not offering me anything?

The book explains that we are often drawn to what is familiar rather than what is good for us. 'As adults, we may then reject potential partners, not because they are wrong, but because they are too well-balanced (too mature, too understanding, too reliable), and their rightness feels unfamiliar and somehow oppressive. We may call these people 'boring' and 'unsexy' and instead head towards people who our unconscious senses will frustrate us in familiar ways. We make mistakes because, deep down, we don't ultimately associate being loved with feeling entirely satisfied.'

Wow. OK.

We may actually fear love and find it easier to put our attention on people who can't love us back, as a clever way of ensuring that we don't end up in a relationship at all. It is easier to endure the pain of unrequited love than it is to 'endure the real demands of love'.

'The fear of love may be motivated by a range of factors, a squeamishness around hope, a self-hatred that makes another person's love feel eerie . . . or a fear of self-revelation which breeds a reluctance to let anyone into the secret parts of ourselves . . .'

This was hitting too close to home. I closed the book, went to the loo and took out my phone.

On Instagram a red-headed life coach had posted: 'The only common denominator in all your failed relationships is YOU! Yes, I know it hurts a little. But it's true – the only common denominator in all your failed relationships is YOU. For years you've been blaming your partners (past and present) for REALLY being the problem. Sadly, I have to let you know . . . it really is you. And I know that's exactly what I had to realize to put my own relationships on a life-changing trajectory to empowerment and success . . .'

No doubt he was trying to sign me up to some course that would show me the error of my way for just $299 or three easy instalments of just $99. I decided to adopt the more tried and tested cure for heartbreak: whiskey in a mug with season two of *Succession*.

The next day I got back to work. Enough of this fucking heartbreak business. Enough relationships. I was asked to write an article about a spiritual teacher called Byron Katie. I said yes, please.

Katie has an approach called The Work, which makes you question everything you think is real. The magazine wanted me to apply her approach to my own life and write about the results. I said yes without considering that what was going on in my life was a broken heart and this article would mean analysing the pain and putting it up for public consumption in 1200 words. Oh well, at least I was getting paid.

Katie's approach is simple. First, she asks us to think of a specific situation where someone upset you. Once an example comes to mind, you write down how you feel about it and don't hold back. Vent. Get all the anger out. This was easy: George had upset me because he was a stone-cold narcissist incapable of love.

With all our hate on the page, Byron Katie invites us to interrogate this belief.

Q1. Is it true? *Yes, it is true – he basically told me he was incapable of love.*

Q2. Can you absolutely know that it's true? (Really take a moment to look at the situation with new eyes in order to be certain that it's true.) *OK, well, it wasn't always true. There were moments of real love between us. He cooked for me, he listened to me.*

Q3. How do you react, what happens, when you believe the first thought? *I feel angry and upset and used and like an idiot for getting involved.*

Q4. Who would you be without that thought? *Free, free to accept that it just hadn't worked out. We'd both tried our best and it wasn't enough.*

Then she invites you to do something called 'Turn It Around', which is where we see how the exact opposite of our original belief might be true. So instead of George being incapable of love . . . was I?

Before I'd even written the Turn-It-Around sentence down, I knew that it was true. I was, in many ways, incapable of love. After all, hadn't I been the one who started things by saying that I didn't want a committed relationship? Hadn't I, in fact, started almost every relationship by telling people that I didn't want to settle down?

George had chosen to walk away and follow his spiritual path – I could relate to that, I had run away time and time again. I related to that feeling of wanting to keep people at a distance. A part of me had always thought that living up a mountain alone was the best solution to life.

George was my mirror. I had gone out with myself. Been dumped by myself. Now I knew what it felt like.

Maybe this is why I avoided relationships: what they showed me about myself was not good. I thought of that line my roommate used on the intimacy retreat: 'I'm the dickhead.'

I thought of Eckhart Tolle's line that relationships are not there to make you happy, they are there to make you 'conscious'.

I texted Hawaiian Santa. 'Is love a shattering of the ego? Is that why I am scared of it?'

'Steady on,' he replied.

The School of Life suggests that instead of fixating on the love interest, or indeed your own flaws, the best way through heartache is to think about what it was that you liked about this person. What were the qualities that attracted you? The chances are, the book says, these qualities will be available in someone else.

So what did I like about him?

Well. I liked having someone to eat with and I liked how intelligent he was and how gorgeous his skin felt and how sensuous he was. I liked having someone to walk around the marshes with. I liked having someone to make love with.

These were absolutely qualities I could find in someone else.

The School of Life also says that the fact that I loved him meant that I could love someone else.

With George, I had opened my heart.

I had allowed myself to want things that I hadn't allowed myself to want before. I wanted someone to talk to, someone to go for walks with, someone to lie in bed next to. These parts of me were a surprise. It surprised me how much I liked having him around, just as it had surprised me how much I'd liked having Daisy around.

I could see that I had also learned enough skills that I was now able to be with someone without losing myself. I didn't go silent the way I had in most of my relationships. I said what was on my mind. This was genuinely new. When we were getting closer, one awkward conversation at a time, I felt like maybe I could do this. Maybe I could hold my own with someone, maybe I could be in a relationship without getting smothered. Maybe I could hear difficult things and speak difficult things. Maybe . . .

'You let yourself fall in love – that's progress!' said Daisy. 'It's something to celebrate.'

Gemma agreed, adding, 'Next time I'd love to see you with someone light-hearted. No more tortured souls trying to save the world.'

The School of Life had one more piece of advice: stop going for people who aren't into you. It's a way of running away from love.

'True love means daring to engage with someone who is available, who thinks, despite our strong background supposition to the contrary, that we are really rather nice.'

Daisy suggested we do some vision boards to mark the new chapter.

I'd done this many times over the years and had usually struggled to put a man on it, with the exception of the guy from Snow Patrol, who went on years earlier after a lot of encouragement from Rachel, and a bottle of red wine. While people around me put down pictures of wedding dresses and hot lovers, I never did. I put pictures of best-selling books and Californian forests, courgettes and people doing yoga. I still hadn't done yoga.

Anyway, this time I put on not one man but three: Lenny Henry (his face looked deep and wise and sad and

soulful – why did I like sad guys?), Keanu Reeves (also deep
and wise and sad and soulful) and a guy off a British show
whose name I can't remember but who looked like he'd know
how to get us down from the mountain alive.

I could look at these men's faces and feel safe. I could see
their goodness.

I also put up pictures of nice living rooms with moss-green
walls and vases of extravagant flowers, leather skirts and silk
blouses and green underwear. Daisy stuck on lots of dollar
signs. It didn't feel very tantric.

After a few hours of sitting on the floor, cutting pictures out
of magazines, I wrote a list of everything I would like in
a man:

Kind
Clever
Funny
Handsome
Tall
Broad shoulders
Solid
Good hands
Good relationship with his family
Stable
Generous
Has a home
Gives to charity
Travels
Encourages me
Listens to me
Thinks I'm beautiful

Calls me out when I'm being a brat
Has his own life

I'd gone from starting the project determined to stay single to writing a shopping list. I didn't know if that was progress or not. My heart was more open, which was good, but I had also become a cliché, which did not feel so good.

But I could picture it for the first time and what's more, I felt like maybe I deserved it, and that such a love could exist, and exist for me.

I could almost touch it now, it was so close.

After a few weeks of online dating it did not feel close.

I hated it. The whole process. The time. The emotional head wreck of it all. The hours of admin, messaging people who would vanish – or being the person who vanishes. Worrying that I was being too fussy or judgemental every time I didn't fancy someone based on a crap picture of them holding a pint, or that I was fundamentally unattractive when the guys I did like didn't like me.

The soul-crushing 'Is this my life?' feeling that came with sitting opposite someone I had nothing in common with in a pub and saying I didn't want another pint but watching as they ordered one for themselves. The beggars-can't-be-choosers pep talk I gave myself when I arranged dates two and three with someone I would never be friends with. The sadness I felt when I realized I was telling myself that I was a beggar. The excitement I felt when I finally met someone I fancied only for them to send a lovely note saying that 'I think you'll agree there was no spark'.

The relief I felt when I looked at the app and it told me I had no new matches and I could just stop.

It brought out all my worst bits. In tantra workshops and festival fields, I could see the beauty in everyone and have deep connections with the most unexpected people, but in dating mode I found myself to be judgemental and box-ticking. What job did they have? What jeans were they wearing? Would my friends like them? Were they tall enough? No doubt they were putting me through the same checklist and I was not passing inspection either.

I tried to remind myself of why it was good to be in a couple, why I was doing this in the first place.

Jan had said that our intimate relationships were the best vehicle for personal growth. Relationships could serve as mirrors, showing us aspects of ourselves that we may not otherwise see. We might not want to see these parts, but in the end it's good for us because it helps us become better people. Alain de Botton says that friends don't always cut it in this regard because mostly they just want to have a nice night with us. Most don't want the hassle of telling us the truth about how deeply flawed we are because, well, it's opening a can of worms that might not get closed before the last tube home.

Within friendships, it's possible to dodge the difficult conversations that you can't avoid in a couple. One friend called the early fights she had with her husband 'formative' because they were making clear what was and wasn't OK, what they could and couldn't live with. Home truths were delivered about one partner's tendency to control, and another's to be reckless with money. She said it wasn't easy hearing that stuff, but it was important. It made her a better person. Him too.

Being in a couple also helps you to learn to compromise

and have difficult conversations, both of which I needed help with.

And it wasn't all about tough love and learning and painful truths being delivered. *Attached* had told me that, as an avoidant, I was depriving myself of love and support and the joy of being part of something bigger than myself. That made sense too.

I thought of Rachel's questions to me about whether it was hard to always be doing everything on my own. I'd said no, because it was the only way I'd known, but I was getting more aware of how tiring it was to be a one-woman band. The joy of seeing George doing the washing up had made me sad and happy in a confusing mixture of ways.

Seeing as Alain de Botton's *Heartbreak* book had made so much sense, I signed up to a class called How to Find Love at The School of Life in Bloomsbury. There were about twenty-five of us in the basement classroom, sitting on office chairs facing towards a man in brown chinos and a jumper. I was sitting next to a woman eating an M&S egg sandwich. I wished she wasn't.

'Who here expects to find a relationship that will make them happy?' the teacher asked.

We all put our hands up and he laughed at us for being idiots. He explained that the idea that relationships should make us happy is a very new concept. Traditionally partnerships had a purpose: to have children, to protect property or to improve our social status. It was only recently that we had started to believe that a romantic partner should give us everything. The romantic myth was created by poets who died at thirty-five and were high on opium, we were told. We laughed. Our high expectations meant that we would always be disappointed. We didn't laugh.

He talked about what might be stopping us from finding love.

First up: our fear of rejection, and a deep fear that if someone really knew us they would run a mile. For some of us that fear meant we rejected people before they could reject us. I was sure I'd done that.

On the flip side, we might also run from partners because we thought we were too good for them. I'd done that too. Quite a lot. He told us that we needed to remember that we, ourselves, were far from perfect and that dating would go a lot better if we could be more generous in our assessments of others. OK, noted.

He ran through some examples of how we might accentuate the positive. So, sure – they might use emojis in their texts, but were they also warm and expressive and trying to make us laugh? And yes, perhaps they did hate their job, but did they have a full and interesting life outside of work?

Finally, we were told something depressing: that we were never going to pick the right person for us.

Great.

In fact, most of us would pick a partner who reminded us of our parents, which meant we would dump someone who was kind and had time for us in favour of a workaholic partner who let us down because it reminded us (unconsciously) of our father.

Or, we might go for someone who was the opposite of our family. If you had a smothering mother, you might (unconsciously) choose someone a bit distant.

And this brought us to the crux of relationships: nobody we picked would be perfect – just as we were not perfect. Our teacher told us that the only way around this was to stop searching for a soulmate and start looking for a 'good enough' partner.

I left the class thinking about the boyfriend I had broken up with in the Tottenham Court Road pub. He was such a good man. His only crime was to like me. I wondered if I met him now whether I'd be better able to handle that. Unfortunately, he was now living with a woman who could also see how good (enough) he was.

On the way to class I had listened to Alain de Botton being interviewed on a podcast.

'I think this constant swiping to find the ideal human is doomed,' he said. He thought that dating apps should let you scroll for a bit and then lock you on a match, and you had to love that person. No excuses. He said that with effort we could find something loveable in everyone and that there was no such thing as the perfect person. Jan said the same – that you could have a successful relationship with anyone if you were both willing, committed and loving.

The Uber driver who took me home from love school might well have been paid by The School of Life. At forty-five – just a couple of years older than me – he was a father of five children and grandfather of two. He had had an arranged marriage at nineteen.

I asked him how that was.

'We found our way. We get on with it. Some days we want to kill each other but we don't. You know?'

'Yeah,' I said. I didn't.

He asked me if I was married – I said I wasn't.

'A lot of people don't realize that nobody is perfect. They don't give love a chance. You know, they go on a date or two, and everyone's got a list in their head. And they start ticking stuff off – but a lot of people are looking for the wrong people. Young girls, they're looking for Mr Right, Mr Six Pack, you know? Those guys are players. And the guys, you know, they want Miss Bikini. But that don't mean nothing.'

'With an arranged marriage you want to make it work – you are in. When I first met my wife I wanted to find all the ways she was good, not all the reasons that she was not good enough. 'Cause I was already committed, you know? With you guys, the way you date, it's like you're all finding reasons for it not to work, thinking of why that person isn't right. Then you end up alone. I have a female friend, your age. Asian lady. We went to school together. We were the first generation born here. So everything was new. We were exploring careers and stuff. Asian girls were wanting their freedom and they ended up making a hell of a lot of money, but they didn't go the marriage route. And now she is crying and depressed all the time. She wishes she had children. But I told her it's never too late, you know, you might not find a spring chicken now – but don't give the old men a miss. Maybe you find someone who is divorced and you can be a stepmum. It's all good. There are ways.'

So this old chicken went on a few more dates and took the 'nobody is perfect' approach. All it did was convince me that I preferred to be single. Yes, I wanted love and sex and silky skin but I did not want to go through this to get it. I was happier alone than trying to force a connection out of thin air, or a message that just said 'Hey . . .'

Maybe I was self-sabotaging, deep down not believing I deserved love. Maybe I was being too fussy and defensive. Maybe I would come to regret not putting in more effort. Or maybe the internet dating thing just didn't work for me.

I would leave it to fate. If someone came along, fine – and if not, also fine. I wasn't giving up, I was trusting.

I went for a walk.

A broad-faced, smiling man walked towards me and I smiled back.

I was smiling back! All the naked workshops had worked! I could now smile at a man in the street! I was a woman of great confidence and sex appeal!

'Can I ask you a question?' he asked as he got closer.

'Yes,' I said, in what I hoped was a flirty way. I liked his big black coat.

'How is your faith?'

Oh.

'My faith in what?'

'In God.'

As I walked away he called after me: 'Don't you want to hear the good news?'

I did not.

16

Mother Love

In the run-up to Christmas, I made a deal with myself: no running off to workshops. No books. No crap dates. No navel-gazing. I was going to nurture what I already had.

I saw Sarah and mum and my sisters. I went for walks. I tidied the flat. It felt good. I even said yes to a party with Rachel.

'I've decided I'm going to do it – I'm going to try to get pregnant on my own,' said Rachel as we got ready at her place. She was wearing a gold jumpsuit with a very low neckline.

'Wow, this is big,' I said.

'Do you think I need tape to make sure these stay in?' she asked, shrugging off the importance of this news.

'Have you got some?'

She said she did and I marvelled at this woman who was so together she had tit tape and a pension.

As I taped her in, she said: 'I'm done with sleeping with the wrong people, trying to make them into the right father. It's stupid. I've been looking at ethical sperm banks.'

'Are there unethical ones?'

'Yeah. This country limits donations to ten families but some don't have limits, so your baby could have hundreds of siblings.'

'Wow.'

'And there have been stories where mental illness hasn't been disclosed—'

'God, I'd never thought of that.'

'Yeah . . . do you think this looks too much?' she said, looking in the mirror.

'You look like a model,' I said. 'If I wasn't as enlightened as I am, I would be annoyed by it. But I am now one with the sisterhood and in touch with my inner beauty, so I'll let it pass.'

She smiled.

'So how does it work? The sperm donor stuff?'

'It's literally like internet dating. You look at their database and pick what you like. I looked for guys with my hair and eye colour – so that the baby is more likely to look like me – and who have decent jobs and degrees. They list their hobbies, and if you pay extra you get details of their personality, celebrity lookalikes—'

'So you can ask for a baby that has a dad who looks like Ryan Gosling?'

'I haven't seen Ryan there but I did see one guy I liked – I'd date him if I saw his profile on an app.'

'What does he look like?'

'They mostly put pictures of the donor as babies, so I don't know what he looks like now, but we have similar colouring and he said really nice things, and the woman on the phone said he made beautiful babies.'

'She actually said that?'

'Yup! And that he was "extremely intelligent".'

'Why he is donating his sperm?'

'He's probably a student trying to make money, but he wrote all the right things – he wrote that the door would always be open to any child that came from this and that any child born to a parent who goes to all this trouble will know they are really loved.'

'He sounds nice,' I said.

'He does,' she said.

'Are you really doing this?' I asked her.

'It looks like it,' she said with a shrug and a smile. 'What about you?' she asked. 'Did you hear from Greg?'

'George. No.'

'You might meet someone at this party.'

'I never meet people at parties.'

'That's the spirit!'

I laughed.

'OK, yes. I might meet someone.'

'Someone normal,' said Rachel. 'No deep feelings or tantric lovers.'

'Yeah, I just want a bit of wham, bam, thank you ma'am.'

We went to the party.

I met a guy. We talked. I liked him. He seemed grown-up. Normal. No necklaces.

'Do you like to be hit?' he asked.

'He asked you that at a party? Straight out?' said Sarah.

We were in the kitchen with remnants of flour and jars of mincemeat. I ate another mince pie out of boredom and topped up our glasses.

'No, he asked me that when we met up for a drink afterwards. At the party he told me that he had just gone through a divorce and was broke. And he asked me if I liked anal sex.'

'At the party?'

'Yes.'

'Then when we met up for a drink—'

'Why did you want to meet him for a drink?'

'I don't know – I liked his honesty.'

'What is it with you and honesty? Didn't some guy tell you that you smelled?'

I laughed.

'Anyway when we met up—'

'Where did you meet?'

'A pub near me. The vegan one.'

'Vegan?'

'Yeah – I don't know what's vegan about it – but anyway, then he asked me if I liked to be hit.'

'And?'

'And I told him that I didn't and he asked me why I didn't like it, and had I really tried it, and was I too much of a control freak to submit? And I said I didn't think I was a control freak and that the whole BDSM thing wasn't something that interested me and he asked me why I'd agreed to go on a date then, and I said I didn't know that was what he liked . . .'

'Fuck this guy! I mean, obviously I hope you didn't . . .?' asked Sarah.

'No, I didn't. He gave me the creeps. In all the tantra stuff it's really important that when you say 'no' it's accepted – it's not a conversation, it's just a 'no' – but this guy, I dunno. It felt like he didn't want to hear the 'no' and I didn't like it.'

'So what happened then?'

'Nothing, I left.'

I didn't really. I stuck around longer than I should have, trying to rescue an uncomfortable conversation. As the date went on, he'd talked about how 'boring' it was when women went on about their weight and how he was done with having 'boring sex' with women who pretended not to want babies but who then changed their minds.

I got the feeling he hated women.

It made me realize the difference between the workshop world and the real world. In the workshop setting I felt totally and utterly safe, and that allowed me to have beautiful experiences. In the real world it didn't always feel so safe.

But I didn't say any of this. I didn't want to bring darkness into the brightly lit kitchen. 'Rachel met someone.'

'That's good.'

'He seemed nice. Quiet and smiley. She looked so good – she was wearing this jumpsuit from Topshop —'

'She always looks good,' said Sarah.

'Yeah, that's true.'

I offered her another pie and she shook her head, pulling up her top to show her tummy. 'I'm Elvis in the Vegas years,' she said. I laughed.

Ella came in looking for more biscuits.

'How many have you had?' Sarah asked.

'Two,' said Ella, her eyes wild with sugar. Sarah raised an eyebrow.

'I did!'

'You can have one more with your programme and then it's time for bed,' she said to Ella.

Ella grabbed it and ran squealing to the living room.

'She's got so grown-up,' I said. I felt guilty that I didn't see her more, that I didn't know her better. 'Thanks for asking me over,' I said.

'It wasn't too boring?'

'No.'

'I can still picture your face at her birthday party . . .'

'What?'

'You looked like you were in hell.'

'Sorry.'

'I know being around a load of kids must be boring,' she said.

'It's not that,' I said. 'I just feel out of place when it's all families . . . like you're all normal and I'm not.'

As I said it I felt impatient with this idea of 'normal' I kept coming back to. What did it even mean? Normal?

'Normal is overrated,' she said looking at the sink full of dishes and debris-covered kitchen counters.

'I spent two hours cleaning this morning, and look at it.' She reached for the wine. 'I've spent my whole life avoiding being a housewife and I am, in fact, a fucking housewife.'

She poured another glass and downed it, filling it up again straight away.

'Dan does way more than most men, but then he comes home and he's like, "Why haven't you done the washing up?" And I'm like, "Are you joking? I'm keeping your child alive."'

She took another swig.

'Marriage is hard. Don't believe anyone when they say it's not. I often think it would be easier if it was just me.'

'Are you two OK?'

She shrugged.

'Are *you* OK?' I asked again.

'Yeah, I'm just tired. I'm always fucking tired. Having a child destroys your life. I mean that literally. It's a total fucking obliteration of the self. I used to travel the world and now I go to Tesco Extra and grab ten minutes in the Costa . . . it was a shit lifestyle choice.'

I laughed, but she didn't.

'You did the right thing not having children. I never thought I'd say that, but you did. If you're not one hundred per cent sure that you want kids, then it's too difficult.'

I didn't say anything.

'We can't fucking afford to have her, that's the reality. Every time some letter comes back from the school about a trip, we have a row. We have no money. Ever. If it wasn't for Steve's dad helping us out we'd be fucked. And I can't see it getting any better.' She topped up our glasses.

'Being a mother is like a prison sentence. It's like that's all I am now. Like until you have kids it's the most important job in the world, and then as soon as you do, nobody gives a shit, you're on your own.'

'Do you regret it? Becoming a mum?' I didn't know if it was OK to ask the question.

'God, no! No. I could never imagine my life without her. I wish I'd started sooner so I could have had more. Which makes no fucking sense because the first six months are awful. You're so alone.'

I felt a pang of guilt. Where had I been during those six months?

'It's like having to run a marathon every day for six months on two hours of sleep. And then biology is fucking crazy 'cause you want to do it again. It makes no sense. None.' She took another drink. 'I love her so much I would die for her – literally. It's mad how extreme it is. I count the minutes until she goes to bed so I finally have some time on my own and then I'm on the sofa looking at pictures of her on my phone.'

I smiled.

'I don't know who I am any more. I don't know what I like, I don't know what I think . . . I look back on my old life and I don't know what I used to do.'

'We used to go to the pub,' I said.

She laughed. 'Can we have a night out soon?' she said.

'Yes,' I said.

'You always say yes, and then you cancel.'

'You cancel too!'

'You cancel more.'

I did. It was true.

'OK. Let's meet in town before Christmas and get day drunk before going to John Lewis.'

'Can we drink after John Lewis too?' she asked.

'Of course.'

'Are you doing any more of those sex weeks?'

'Yeah, I hope so. I love it, it's been a really important thing in my life.' It felt good to say that and to not make a joke about it.

I waited for a snarky comment but it didn't come.

'Why was it important?' she asked.

'I don't know, I guess I just needed help in figuring out how to have relationships and overcoming some shame around sex . . . and now, well – I dunno, now the people I know through tantra are my friends, and I like being with them.'

'I wish I could do it,' she said.

I was shocked.

'Do you? I thought you hated the idea.'

'No, why did you think that?'

'I dunno, I just thought you thought it was really weird.'

'No – I thought you were being weird about it and not telling me what happened,' she said. 'You do all these things and meet new people, while I'm . . .' She looked around the room. 'Here. And you never ask me to do anything with you any more, you never call—'

'I never know the right time to call, you have so much on —'

'Call any time! I don't want to spend my life with all these mum friends – I want to see my real friends. I want to see you.'

'I feel like you think what I'm doing is stupid while you're living a proper grown-up life . . .'

'What's grown-up about spending all night cleaning up sick?'

'I dunno. It's just that's what we should be doing at this age,' I said.

'Says who?' she asked.

'I dunno!'

I could see that I had projected my own shame onto my friends. I imagined that they were judging me, when really it was *me* judging me. I had felt ashamed of being single, with hang-ups around sex and hand-jobs. I felt ashamed of my tiny rented flat.

But I wasn't ashamed any more – I was proud of having done tantra, of having the courage to explore an area that terrified me, of going back to school to learn things I'd never been taught. That was nothing to be ashamed about – it was something to brag about, in *Pussy* terms. And as for my tiny flat, I could hardly keep that clean, so god knows how I'd cope in a proper house.

As I walked up the stairs to go to the loo, I felt glad that I'd set up my life the way I had. I was exhausted even thinking about Sarah's. But I still wondered if mine was immature. As a forty-something woman, I was still someone's child, not someone's mother. Sarah and Gemma had passed over a threshold that I had not. They had moved from being the picture to the frame.

On the loo, I looked into the bath, with its leftover water with a blue duck bobbing in it. I had a flashback of being in the bath with my sister, making Mohicans in our hair with shampoo bubbles, our skinny white knees sticking up out of the water. I remembered mum picking us up out of the water and wrapping us in a towel, hugging us as she rubbed us dry.

For the first time it hit me – the thousands of hours of work and love and care and cleaning and exhaustion and fights and kisses that mum had given us. Hours that I didn't even remember. Hours that were money in the bank of security I had been unwittingly drawing on all my life.

I had never thanked her for any of it. Not really. Not enough.

I stood in the corridor watching Sarah reading to her daughter. She was lying down next to Ella, whose little head was leaning into her mum's shoulder, her face looking at the book in rapt attention. Sarah turned the page and did a funny voice. Ella burst into giggles and gazed up at her mum.

She beamed with joy.

Sarah's exhausted face beamed right back.

I spent the next day in bed feeling joyfully child-free, watching episodes of *Queer Eye*. In one of the episodes, the show's experts were making over a middle-aged high-school teacher who had dedicated her life to her family and her pupils, and had been wearing the same jeans for twenty years.

'I just think it's how my generation was raised,' she was explaining to the boys. 'We just sort of skipped that chapter of me. When you think about yourself, you're being selfish. And being selfish is, like, a very bad thing – in my generation, you know?'

'I don't want you to skip the chapter of you any more,' one of the presenters said, before cutting off her fiery red mullet.

Mum, it seemed, was also re-writing her role by refusing to cook Christmas lunch for the first time in forty years.

'I'm on a Christmas sabbatical,' she announced as we walked to The Elderfield pub for a singalong of Christmas carols.

'What?'

'We're going to Michelle's this year. I don't want to cook. And I'm not going to bother with a cake or pudding.'

'What? No way! Mum.'

'None of you like pudding, and I'm the only one who eats the cake.'

'That's not true – I love pudding and I eat the cake, I just wish you wouldn't put so much marzipan on it.'

We'd gone early but the pub was already packed. We found stools by the bar. Mum took off her coat to show a pink-and-gold striped top.

'Is that a new top?' I asked.

'Yes, do you like it?'

'I've never seen you wear that colour before.'

'I thought I'd try something new. From you-know-where.'

You-know-where was TK Maxx. Always TK Maxx.

She wiggled on the stool, singing along with *Dashing through the snow, in a one-horse open sleigh . . .*'

Who was she? This woman wearing pink for the first time in her life, in a pub . . . singing and wiggling?

She smiled and waved at a young couple across the bar.

'Who are they?' I asked.

'My neighbours,' she said.

They came over.

'Your mom is amazing,' Caitlin said to me while mum was chatting to her partner.

'Is she?' I asked. I looked at her. For a second she didn't look like my mum. She looked so young and pretty. I imagined her in pubs years before me and my sisters arrived, chatting, flirting, being free. A whole other person. Her own person . . . I felt irrationally irritated.

'I miss mine,' said Caitlin. 'She's in Australia.'

After a couple of hours of singing and drinking, I walked her home. She told me off for not wearing a scarf.

'You'll get sick,' she said.

I felt irritated again. I was in my forties. I was capable of deciding whether to wear a scarf or not. But then, I was in my forties and still wanted my mum to make me a Christmas cake. The concept of making it myself hadn't even entered my head.

We kept walking.

'Please make a cake and I'll buy a pudding.'

'You can't buy a pudding, they'll be horrible.'

'No they're nice – I'll get one of those fancy Waitrose ones. I'll google which is the best. Please.'

'I'll think about it.'

'OK.'

We kept walking, past the bookshop on Lower Clapton Road. We stopped to look in the window.

'*Tomorrow Sex Will be Good Again*,' she said, reading one of the book titles out loud. She paused for half a second. 'I doubt it,' she said and carried on walking.

'And I'm not putting up a tree.'

'What?'

On Christmas Day we went to our cousin Michelle's and sat around a table of friends and family, sixteen of us. Daisy was there too, and smiled politely as Michelle went into great detail about how she had cooked the bird. I was about to remind Michelle that Daisy was vegetarian but Daisy shook her head and mouthed, 'It's fine,' and kept smiling and nodding.

'It smells amazing,' she said, handing out the presents she'd bought everyone. I'd told her not to but she didn't want to come empty-handed. There were bottles of fizz, even though she didn't drink, and boxes of chocolates and presents for the kids.

'Are you sure it's OK for me to join?' she'd kept asking before the day.

'Yeah, of course it is. The more the merrier.'

'Are you sure?' she'd asked again when she stayed on the blow-up bed in the kitchen on Christmas Eve.

'Michelle loves having people over. And having someone who isn't family will make us behave better. Please come.'

The day flew by, and it ended with everyone – mum included – dancing to Prince by the fire at midnight.

She did make a cake in the end. It was delicious. I put a photo of it on Instagram.

'You have ten likes, mum.'

'Is that good?'

'You haven't gone viral.'

'But have I gone bacterial?' she asked.

At one point when mum was dancing with her paper hat on and Michelle was topping up our glasses, I saw Daisy sitting on the sofa, gazing at the scene as if she was watching a Hallmark movie.

'That was the best Christmas ever,' she said when we were back at mine, sitting in fleecy pyjamas on the sofa.

'Really?' I asked.

'Your family is great.'

'Are they?' I asked.

'Yes,' she said, and her tone was serious.

'You walk into a room and you don't see it, but your mum's eyes light up . . . I've never had that. I've never been the most important person in a room. I know that you think I'm stupid going after all the wrong guys. But I just want to matter to someone. I just want a home.'

I felt a pain in my chest when she said this. I *had* judged her, going from one man to the next. I'd got frustrated that she put all her hopes in strangers, people who were not good enough for her. I'd never once seen what was driving her behaviour: she was trying to get a love and safety she'd never had as a child. A love and safety she deserved and needed.

A love and safety that I had never spent a minute of my life without.

I thought of how many times I'd moved back to mum's in between jobs and mini breakdowns, or how many times I'd been fed and loved by my aunties and cousins, always welcomed with open arms and the words, 'Stay as long as you like.'

It meant I could never fall far. There was always someone to catch me. This was why I could be so free and easy with romantic partnerships – I wasn't looking for love and security from a partner – I already had so much of it in my family.

In that moment I saw that having a loving, supportive family – especially a mother – was the single biggest privilege any human could have. The greatest love. All this time looking for love, and I was swimming in a river of it all along.

Daisy had never had that.

'You matter to me,' I said.

And I realized as I said it that there weren't many people I wanted to commit to, but I wanted to commit to Daisy.

'Could I be your family?' I asked.

'I don't want to be too much,' she stammered.

'You're not too much,' I said, and I meant it. I often found people too much. I felt the pressure of people's needs. I was too quick to go into rescuer mode and to feel guilty when I couldn't do what I thought was enough. But with Daisy I never felt any pressure, never felt any guilt. I wanted to be there for her.

She looked at me, her Disney-princess-eyelinered eyes looking impossibly huge as I said: 'I know it's not a ring, or a dress, but I want you to know that as long as I live, you will have a home.'

———

For New Year, Daisy went on a yoga retreat and I stayed home alone, going to bed at 9 p.m. and waking up to the sound of fireworks. I opened the blinds in my bedroom and watched the showers of light from my bed. I checked my phone. I got a text from the Greek, wishing me happy new year. I wished him a happy new year back and then fell asleep.

In the morning I went through all the messages I'd been sent in the small hours. There was another one from the Greek. He told me he was coming over to London for his godchild's christening. I left a voice note for Daisy telling her the news.

She called me right back. 'You have to give him the best lingam massage of his life!'

'I'm still shit at those. Anyway, how are you? How's it going? Have you met anyone nice?'

'Yes!'

'Who is he?'

'She.'

'Oh!'

'I can't talk now but keep me posted on the Greek.'

When we hung up she sent me a link from Layla Martin's site: 'How to give mind-blowing hand-jobs.' I started watching the video, then stopped. How much time was I going to spend trying to learn how to be good enough for men? How much time had I spent reading books and trying to improve myself? Maybe I didn't need to learn any tricks, maybe I was OK with my sweaty hands and sexual insecurities.

My mind started to go down the usual 'you're fat' road, but I stopped myself.

No, Marianne. No. Enough.

I wondered whether to book a wax, to subject myself to the socially acceptable torture that women had to undergo in order to be, well, socially accepted.

I didn't. He could take me as I was.

17

True Love

The Greek had booked a fancy hotel for two nights.

He had already checked in and gone to meet his friend by the time I arrived. He told me to pick up a room key at reception. I walked into the huge room with a bed the size of a ship. I saw folded copies of the *FT* and *The Economist* on the table. His bag was in the corner and a couple of shirts were hanging up in the wardrobe. His presence was in the room, and I liked it.

I'd thrown out the peephole undies I'd bought to see him last time – they were never me. They'd been replaced by a pretty lace bra that did not make my boobs look like they were being held hostage. They went into a drawer.

I went down to the bar and sat by the fire. I was messaging Gemma pictures of the art when he walked in through the back of the bar. My heart leapt, and I stood up from the sunken sofa.

'Hello!'

'Hello!'

He gave me a bear hug, squeezing me tight and lifting me up off the ground.

'Stop, you'll break your back!' I said. 'Welcome back to London.'

He looked smiley and handsome, and I was reminded

again of why I'd fancied him the first time I saw him in the
coffee shop.

We sat down and I went into a flurry of small talk.

I was on autopilot – filling the silences, talking my way
over any nerves, like it was no big deal that he was here
in London and that we were in a hotel. Obliterating intimacy . . . had I learned nothing?

He asked if I'd got into the room OK.

'Yeah, it's gorgeous.' I had been worried about him spending so much and wanted to offer to split it, but Gemma told
me not to. He was making a gesture and I should accept it
generously.

'Can I get us dinner to say thank you?' I asked. He said yes
and over steak and chips we talked about his work, the Greek
economy and the environment. After dinner we walked back
to the hotel. He reached for my hand and I let him hold it.

When we got into the room, he went to the bathroom and
I sat on the bed and put the television on. An actress from
Game of Thrones was sitting on Graham Norton's sofa next to
a comedian whose name I couldn't remember. I felt nervous
to be in a hotel room with the Greek. Television, as always,
would distract me.

When he came out of the bathroom he was wearing a thick
towelling bathrobe with the hotel's name across the chest.

'Are you OK?' I asked him.

'Last time we met we didn't even kiss.'

'I know.'

'I regret that.'

'It can be remedied,' I said.

I turned the television off.

I was always looking for men to make the first move, but
this time I did. This wasn't about me being picked or chosen
or *approved of*. And it didn't matter what moves I had or didn't

have – all that mattered was that I cared about this man. This man who I'd walked up to in a coffee shop years earlier. This man who spent his life loving others in the realest, messiest and most exhausting way. I wanted to give him something back.

Since going to The School of Life, I had read everything Alain de Botton had written about relationships.

I read a post which explained that most of us have a childlike vision of love. Ideally we grew up with parents who gave us love and looked after us, and it was never our job to ask them about their day or to let them have a tantrum. It was all coming one way. And as adults, a part of us still wants it to be like that. We think of love in terms of getting love – not giving it.

German psychoanalyst Eric Fromm agrees. I'd bought his book *The Art of Loving* and underlined this passage: 'Most people see the problem of love primarily as that of being loved, rather than that of loving, of one's capacity to love. Hence the problem to them is how to be loved, how to be lovable. In pursuit of this aim they follow several paths. One, which is especially used by men, is to be successful, to be as powerful and rich as the social margin of one's position permits. Another, used especially by women, is to make oneself attractive, by cultivating one's body, dress, etc . . .'

I had probably spent a lot of my life trying to be 'loveable' – cultivating my appearance, smiling nicely, people-pleasing. I had written shopping lists – literally – of what I wanted from a man. But had I ever written a shopping list of what I could give him?

When I first went to Athens, I went there wanting to 'get' love. I wanted a good story to bring home. I wanted another adventure to add to my life. When it came to my romantic relationships I think I was often in 'getting' mode – getting validation, getting attention.

Eric Fromm says: 'Infantile love follows the principle: "I love because I am loved." Mature love follows the principle: "I am loved because I love." ' In other words, love is not a feeling, it is an action.

It was time to mature when it came to love. To treat love as a verb, not an acquisition. To give love rather than to seek it.

We woke up to his alarm. He jumped up in a panic.

'Everything OK?' I asked.

'Yes, it's OK – it's the alarm for my dad's medication, I forgot to switch it off.'

We ordered breakfast in bed and I felt the weight he was carrying.

'You look like a painting,' he said, and it seemed to make him sad.

That afternoon we walked around London and went to galleries and sat in coffee shops. It felt easy to be with him. He talked about art and politics and his memories of London, and I loved to listen to him. I loved his mind. I pictured us living together in London, doing these things all the time and for the first time in my life the idea didn't fill me with panic. It would be nice, actually. But neither was I clinging to it. It was just a little vision that floated in and floated out again.

We went to the theatre and had room service when we got back.

I told him about the tantra and everything I'd learned, how I found it hard to commit to people and had a lot of fear around sex. It felt embarrassing to say this stuff to him, but as he had done since our first conversation, I felt he understood me in a way that few people did.

'It's logical for women to be scared of sex,' he said. 'For most of history sex could result in pregnancy, which could result in death. Or it could lead to being shamed or isolated . . . so it makes perfect sense for there to be fear.'

I'd never thought of that before. Through his eyes my fears were not shameful, they were perfectly rational.

We talked about relationships and I told him that I didn't seem to be able to do them in the way that others did, and he said he was the same.

'I find it hard to connect,' he said.

'I've never felt that you had that problem,' I said.

The thought occurred to me again that I'd spent so much time looking at my own insecurities, my own avoidance, I didn't see that other people had their issues too.

I woke up the next morning to the sound of him closing his suitcase.

'What time is it?' I asked.

'It's nine, I need to go,' he said.

'Really?'

'The christening is in an hour.'

I started to get up.

'No, stay in bed, you have another couple of hours until check-out.'

He leaned down to hug me. He gripped me like a vice.

And then he vanished.

'Don't you want to run after him?' Daisy asked, when I texted her from the hotel bed after he'd left.

The thought honestly hadn't occurred to me.

As I sat up against the puffy headboard, alone in a hotel

room, I thought of a writing seminar I'd done with Robert McKee. He was this big-deal teacher who travelled the world lecturing, charging hundreds for students to sit in freezing cold rooms learning the structure of stories.

He argued that there were no great love stories any more because young people were incapable of sacrifice. He'd said something along the lines of nowadays, if someone wanted you to go off into the sunset with them, you'd pass because you were up for promotion.

'It's true,' I'd said to my sister afterwards. 'I wouldn't drop everything for a man.'

'You consider yourself to be young, do you?' she'd said.

But young or old, I had never felt the urge to quit my life and follow a man around the world, just as I hadn't felt the need to quit my life to follow a friend around the world, or my sister for that matter. Why was it that if I followed my sister to New York it would be odd, but to do the same for a man was romantic? Even if it ended up in heartbreak and expensive flights home two months later?

And did love have to involve self-sacrifice as the story guru had suggested? Was it a sign of selfishness that I had no interest in self-sacrifice? Hadn't women done enough of that? This man, who got paid a lot of money to travel the world talking about love, what sacrifices had he made? Or was it always the wife who was expected to do that?

Maybe there weren't answers to these questions.

All I knew was that I was glad I'd had those days with the Greek. Not because I thought it was going to lead to any kind of happy ever after, but because it was a way for us to be happy right now. But I realized something else as well: I was also glad to be here now, alone. To be a woman, alone in a hotel room, thinking about love.

What a privilege.

'Paradoxically, the ability to be alone is the condition for the ability to love,' Fromm says.

I didn't want to leave.

I looked up the prices to stay another night and was shocked. Mum would kill me if I booked a night in a London hotel when my flat was half an hour's tube ride away. But why should fancy mini-breaks and hotels only be reserved for those in couples? Why couldn't I romance myself?

I rang down and asked about availability. The man told me the place was quiet and that they could give me a good deal. When I hung up I squealed with excitement and kicked my feet up and down on the fancy bed. I knew Regena Thomas-hauer would approve of the act of self-love, as much as mum wouldn't.

That afternoon I ordered room service and watched trash TV while eating a fancy beef burger which came under a silver dome, next to heavy cutlery wrapped inside a linen napkin. I ate the burger with relish, enjoying the juice, the meat, the flavour. I dipped each of the skinny chips into a tiny silver bowl of mayonnaise, and washed it down with a glass of red. This was it. This was living.

I left the tray in the corridor and went to the bathroom – which was the size of my flat – and ran a bath. I poured all the tiny bottles of Molten Brown into the water and watched them bubble into mountains of froth before stepping in.

As I lay in the warm water, made silky with the bath oils, a glass of red on the tiled floor and Eric Fromm's book folded open on the closed loo, I had the thought: *this* is the woman I was meant to be.

This woman, here, alone in a hotel room with the whole city at her feet. This woman with the company of her thoughts, a book and a bath . . . This woman with total freedom.

Hours earlier, I had loved and been loved as best as either of us were able to – and now I was on my own, happy.

I wanted both: the togetherness and the solitude.

And I had it.

Over the last few months I had taken down the walls I had built to keep out love. I'd faced my fear of sex, my fear of men, my fear of intimacy and my fear of commitment. I'd almost faced my fear of conflict and of saying no to people, and was beginning to make progress with boundaries. Well, I mean, at least I knew what boundaries were now.

I'd learned to embrace my sexuality and to drop the deep, dark, gnarly shame I didn't know I'd had about being a woman. I had opened my heart to love and said those three words to another and even if they had not been said back, it felt important to say them.

But now I really wanted to say them to myself.

Because, alone in a London hotel room in a fancy bath with fancy oils, I did love myself.

'I love you,' I said out loud, and laughed at the silliness and the relief of it.

And if I was sitting in this bath in love with myself, that meant that I had to be in love with everything that had happened to get me here – all the years of feeling inadequate and a weirdo single freak. They were not a mistake, they were all part of what had brought me to this moment. Which I would not change for anything.

I realized that for all the time spent examining the ways in which I seemed to be lacking, I never gave much thought to the things that I could and did do. How utterly rich and full of love my life had been. I thought of the travel and adventures I'd had – the planes I'd got on, the interesting people I'd met, the hotel rooms I'd been in on my own, thrilled with the independence and glamour of my life. Perhaps my ability to enjoy things alone was not a character flaw – perhaps it was a gift?

As a single woman, I've lived my life with an echo of 'What's wrong with me?' inside my head. It's followed me every day. What's wrong with me that men don't like me? What's wrong with me that when they do, I don't like them? What's wrong with me that I don't seem to want the thing that everyone around me wants? What's wrong with me that I have none of the trappings of adult life? What's wrong with me?

At that moment the truth was clear. Nothing was wrong.

Gemma came to visit a week later. I told her all about the Greek and the hotel and getting room service on my own. I told her about the realization that I had become the woman I'd always wanted to be.

'You were always that woman to me,' she replied instantly.

According to Irish priest turned poet John O' Donohue, 'A friend is a loved one who awakens your life in order to free the wild possibilities within you . . . The one you love, your *anam cara*, your soul friend, is the truest mirror to reflect your soul. The honesty and clarity of true friendship also brings out the real contour of your spirit.'

Gemma was my soul friend.

Our friendship had given me so much of what romance had promised and never delivered. She was the fire to my water. The get-up-and-go to my sit-down-and-sleep.

In many ways, Gemma had shown me how to love.

The first meal she'd cooked for me, in her flatshare in Dublin, was a Thai curry. She'd put the rice into a cup and turned it upside down so that it made a little dome. To me this was the height of sophistication.

The food was delicious. 'It was made with love,' she'd said. Made with love? What the hell did that mean? Having spent fifteen years by her side, I now knew what it meant. Gemma did everything – cook, parent, work, chat – with love. She loved as a verb.

I thought about how we devalue friendships – we say that we're 'just' friends. What was 'just' about it? What was inconsequential about witnessing someone's life for fifteen years? Fifteen years of loving, listening, laughing and looking out for someone? Drying their tears after yet another disappointment, cheering each other on through every new adventure?

I thought of Alain de Botton's idea that love means helping the other person to be a better version of themselves. She did that with me. She said things that I didn't want to hear but she said them anyway for my own good. She believed in me in ways that I didn't believe in myself.

If you're a single woman, friendship is presented as a consolation prize. But friendship isn't a consolation prize. For me, it had been the real thing. I'd read somewhere that the word friend and 'free' came from the same origin. That made sense. The freedom of friendship was what worked for me. There was no contract, just a choice every day to stay in each other's lives.

I thought of the pressure we put on The One to be a certain way – to look a certain way, act a certain way. I thought of the shopping list I'd written at New Year. I never wrote these kinds of lists for friends. I didn't have an idea of what a 'best friend' needed to look like. We let each other be who we were, without trying to make the other fit into any mould. We adored, endured and forgave each other.

None of that was to say it was perfect. Of course it wasn't. Female friendship is often portrayed as a sugar-coated love. But it wasn't sugar-coated – it was messy and challenging. I thought of Jan saying that if you couldn't handle conflict you couldn't have a close relationship. I still had a lot of work to do around that, but my friendships had allowed me to take baby steps.

After a day of shopping and a boozy lunch, we came back to mine. 'Shall we watch *Sex and the City* for old time's sake?' I asked. We used to watch hours of the show together in our late twenties.

On my laptop screen, Gemma and I caught up with Samantha, Miranda and Charlotte at a birthday dinner for Carrie in a diner. Carrie was bemoaning that she was thirty-five and alone. I rolled my eyes. Thirty-five. A mere baby.

Miranda responded: 'You're not alone,' and Carrie said she knew she had them, but was sad about not having a boyfriend in her life . . . much less a soulmate.

Charlotte's face did that thing it did when she was about to pipe up, and then she came out with this classic line: 'Maybe our girlfriends are our soulmates,' she said. 'And guys are just people to have fun with.'

Then it hit me.

'You've been the love of my life,' I tell Gemma.

She turned to me in surprise.

'I don't know what I did to deserve that,' she said.

'It's just the way it is,' and as I said it I felt the familiar painful swell in my chest that came from declaring my true feelings.

She reached for my hand, and we looked back at the screen.

When she left the next evening, I sat at my desk looking out the window at the chip shop. Behind it, the sun was setting streaky orange and purple.

I thought about all the love I'd shared with friends, all the romantic moments. I remembered slow dancing on a rainy night in Soho with Sarah as a busker sang Nina Simone's 'My

Baby Just Cares for Me'. I remembered Daisy showing up at my front door with flowers when dad died and Rachel sending me the book on heartbreak, knowing I'd be too proud to buy it myself.

All those years of people asking me if I was seeing anyone, I wish I'd said, 'Yes, I'm seeing several people and they are all amazing. I don't live with them and I don't have sex with them but they are the loves of my life. I am so lucky.'

I checked Instagram and saw a post by sweary self-help author Mark Manson.

It said: 'You are going to be single for the rest of your life. How do you feel?'

Then the next slide: 'You will have no friends for the rest of your life. How do you feel?'

Well, that would be unbearable.

18

Maybe, Baby

'Did you see the article on this in the paper?'

'No.'

'It's about how women don't want to have children.'

'Right.'

'I have it here somewhere,' mum said, looking on the table next to the sofa, where her old newspapers were folded, crosswords facing up. 'I kept it for you.'

She rummaged until she found it and flicked through the pages.

'Here it is. Apparently in Hungary the fertility rate has plunged to 1.49 live births per female.'

'Point four nine?' I repeated, unable to get my head around what 0.49 of a baby was.

'In Sweden it's 1.85, Denmark 1.76 and Iceland 1.75.'

'Hmm.'

Mum read from the piece: '"The problem is not lack of sex, it's pesky women: they just don't want babies any more. Well, maybe one – the only child is becoming the norm – but seldom more than two. A fifth of British women in their forties are now childless. Or, as many would put it, child-free".'

'A fifth?' I repeated. I didn't know if that sounded like a lot or not a lot.

Mum kept reading: '"Indeed, modernity has uncovered a

strange truth: that when women, regardless of culture, religion or race, get the chance to have fewer kids, they seize it. Women, it seems, do not naturally glory in motherhood; they see pregnancy as frightening, painful, even life-threatening; they realize raising small children makes you vulnerable, financially dependent on men or the state. It's boring and exhausting . . ."'

I was sure Gemma did not see motherhood this way. I wondered if Sarah did.

'Apparently South Korea has the world's lowest birth rate at 0.88,' said mum, reading aloud again. 'Korean women have no appetite for unpaid domestic drudgery. They even have a word for it – "sampo" – meaning to relinquish relationships, marriage and children . . .'

'Huh,' I said, repeating 'sampo' in my head. It sounded nice.

Mum continued: '"When asked to choose between career and family, women increasingly choose work . . . Only nations who combine poverty with extreme gender inequality have spiralling populations, such as Somalia (6.02) or Niger (6.9). Sub-Saharan Africa is projected to double in size by 2050. Yet the Gates Foundation estimates that there are 220 million women in developing countries who don't want to get pregnant but lack access to birth control . . ."' Mum put the paper down. 'I always remember my mother saying that she would never have had the number of children she had if —'

'If what?'

'If there was a way of avoiding it. As it was she had eight pregnancies, bless her.'

She'd had seven children and one baby that died when he was just ten months old. She was not allowed to go to the funeral. She'd watched as the tiny white coffin had passed outside her sitting room window. She went on to have four more children. There was no contraception and even when it was available it was forbidden by the Church.

'She was a frustrated businesswoman. She came alive when she was involved in something. She ran the farm and a guest-house in the summer. She was always coming up with ways to earn extra money. How many women are there like that in their houses? And how many really feel like it's their sole purpose to have kids?'

'Yeah, but it doesn't have to be your sole purpose now – you can have kids and keep your career.'

'That's what suits some people, but it's not what suits everybody. You talk about feminism – feminism is women having the freedom to choose whatever it is they want. When my mother was growing up, getting married was pretty much your only option in life. But you have options and opportun-ities . . . Some people desperately want to have children and if they can't they go to the ends of the earth and spend thou-sands to make it happen. That's how they're made. But it's not like that for everyone and it shouldn't be. Nobody should tell you how to live your life, or make you feel guilty if you've decided to have twenty kids or no kids . . . I never thought "I can't wait to be a mother". I was looking after children from the age I could stand. Being a mother was never my dream, and it's all I've done. Until your father got sick and I went back to work, and that was the best thing that could have happened.'

I remember that so clearly – mum being terrified of going back into the classroom after twenty-five years out of work. She was so stressed – by the new work environment and the new technology – that she fainted during her first week. But she didn't give up, and she eventually became the most

sought-after supply teacher in the area. The kids called her
'Mrs Powerful'.

'I don't think you'd be able to do the work you do and have
a family,' she said.

'Some people do.'

'Yes, of course – but it would be hard. Children literally take
every minute of your day. It's exhausting. It's not for everyone. You don't know who you are or what you are – there's
always someone needing something from you – something to
eat, something to be cleaned . . . you're a glorified servant,'
said mum. She continued: 'There are so many times you wish
you could shut the door for a couple of days and have nothing
to do with them. Every mother has that. You wish to God you
had time for yourself. I remember you used to wait outside
the toilet for me . . .'

I remembered that too. Knocking on the door, asking how
much longer she'd be. Not because we wanted to use the
toilet but because we wanted her. We wanted every bit of her.
Constantly. And she gave it.

There was not a minute of the day she wasn't there for
us. We didn't go a day without anything – food, love, security, routine, clean clothes . . . She dropped us to school, she
picked us up, she had dinner made every evening and we
moaned that it wasn't what we wanted. She washed our hair
and cleaned our clothes, she listened to every schoolyard
drama and helped us with our spellings.

She was never, ever not there. Ever.

And I don't know how happy it made her.

As children, we'd ask her everything: what was her favourite colour? (blue); what was her favourite meal? (bacon and
cabbage); did she think there was a heaven? (didn't know);
what was it like when she was a child? (different).

And then we'd ask her when was the best time in her life.

She would light up when she talked about living in Dublin in her twenties. She was a teacher with enough money to pay the bills and buy nice clothes. She had her own car, her independence, and she could spend all weekend reading in bed . . .

Whenever we asked her about when she was happiest, it was these times she talked about – before dad, before us.

'What would you have done if you didn't have children?' I asked.

'I'd have travelled, had a career, been free,' she said.

It hit me then that I was living my mother's un-lived life.

Sheila Heti's book says, 'Maybe motherhood means honouring one's mother.' Maybe not choosing motherhood was honouring her, too.

Two weeks later, I paid a man with icy hands to put his piano fingers inside me. I gasped with the shock and the pain as he placed a balloon inside my uterus and inflated it.

Shortly afterwards, I was in a Harley Street waiting room, waiting to find out if I was fertile.

I braced myself for the likelihood that I'd left it too late and that after years of working and drinking and stressing, my fertility was gone. I prepared myself for the moment he told me that, and I realized I'd been fooling myself when I said I didn't want kids. I braced myself for the heartbreak I would feel as the weight of a lost life came crashing down on me.

It didn't happen like that.

A man with expensive-looking hair and skin beckoned me into a high-ceilinged room where he stood behind a mahogany desk the size of my kitchen.

'Miss Power,' he said, gesturing to the seat.

He picked up papers and talked about eggs and follicles. It meant nothing to me.

'The upshot,' he said, 'is that you are very fertile for someone of your age.'

'Oh.'

'Unusually fertile, I would say.'

'Oh, right.'

He smiled at me and I felt a swell of pride. I was a woman! A real woman! A fertile woman! For a second, I allowed myself to imagine that I was an entirely different person to the one I was – a person who would fall in love, settle down and have a baby. A 'normal' person. A wife. A mother. A 'good' woman.

But I wasn't that person. I knew that. For better or worse, I just wasn't.

He looked at me, waiting for a reaction. I thought of how many women would give anything to be told this news.

'Of course, with your age, there isn't time to spare, but the results are positive,' he reiterated.

'Thank you so much,' I said.

My second feeling was guilt. What a waste. What a waste to have all this working equipment and not want to use it.

I thought of Rachel.

It didn't seem fair.

I had no doubts this time.

Not one.

Motherhood was not for me.

I was in awe of how Sarah and Gemma were raising their kids. Genuinely in awe. The love they gave their children, the patience, the way they listened to them . . . how much they enjoyed their company and the energy they had even on a couple of hours of broken sleep. I could not do what they did.

I slept a good eight hours a night and got every cold going. As an up-and-down moody type, being with others for too long made me cranky and exhausted. Family life was 24/7 with others. As for the rigours of domesticity, they were not my strength.

But while these were explanations, I didn't think they were the reasons why I didn't want children. I wasn't sure there was a reason. It just wasn't something I wanted.

It wasn't that I was prioritizing my career or that I wanted to travel. It wasn't because I didn't want to give birth – although I didn't. It wasn't because I didn't think I'd be a good mum. Actually, I thought I'd be a great mum, as my mum had been to me, and her mum had been to her. I'd give it my all, but that's what it would be: my all. There would be nothing left of me.

I remembered watching *The Hours* when it first came out. There was a scene in which Julianne Moore's character, a 1950s suburban mum, left her child and checked into a hotel with sleeping pills, intent on ending a life of stifling domesticity and sexual repression. I was twenty-five when I watched it, and I remember thinking: that would be me.

I'd seen something on Instagram once that asked: 'What suffering are you most suited to?' For me, it was not that suffering.

It was only once I'd had the fertility test that I started reading about women who forego motherhood. I saw myself in the essays in *Selfish, Shallow, and Self-Absorbed: Sixteen Writers on the Decision Not to Have Kids*, edited by Meghan Daum. I felt vindicated by the book *Beyond Motherhood: Choosing a Life Without Children* by Jeanne Safer. In the introduction she writes, 'My decision never to bear children reflects my entire history, that interaction of temperament and circumstance, fear and desire, capacities and limitations, that makes me who I am.'

Exactly. I didn't even consciously know or understand all the factors that had gone into making me a woman who didn't want children, but I didn't really need to understand them. It was just how I was.

I phoned Daisy to tell her about the tests.

'I think I'll mother in other ways,' I found myself saying.

'You've been a very good mother to me,' she said.

And so it was that I decided that I'd end my explorations of love. I had everything I needed and wanted: friends, family, singledom and sexual liberation. I even had true love and an (adult) child. What more could I want? There was nothing to change about my life. Nothing missing. Nothing more that I needed.

And then lockdown happened.

19

I'm Going to Die Alone

I used to watch scenes on TV where people were put into solitary confinement and I'd think I could do that. I thought I'd meditate, sleep and write, and I honestly couldn't see what the fuss was about.

I used to listen to *Desert Island Discs* and when Kirsty asked some mega-successful person about how they'd fare on their own, and the mega-successful person admitted they would struggle, I'd think: 'LOSER! You might be the world's leading cancer surgeon who has also started an academy for under-privileged kids and writes poetry on the side, but deep down you are weak and needy and I am not! I would be just fine on a desert island! Take that, you MBE genius!'

But as Covid-19 put the world into lockdown, it seemed that the independence I had prided myself on was a sham. Faced with a real-life emergency, all I wanted to do was cling to another human. Any human. I felt panicked – genuinely panicked – on my own.

I bitterly regretted every life choice I'd ever made that had resulted in me alone in a one-bedroom flat in the middle of a global pandemic. I regretted anyone I'd ever broken up with. My aloneness felt like a punishment for my arrogance and immaturity, fussiness and selfishness. I would have given any-thing to have someone on the sofa with me. The song 'You Might Need Somebody' went around and around in my head.

This is why people are in couples, I thought. For the first time I really, really got it. It wasn't anything to do with societal expectations or fancy wedding days, it was a basic human need to be close to one another.

Until now, my friends and family provided all the insulation I needed. Now they didn't. They were hunkering down in their units. Daisy was having 'olympic' lovemaking sessions with her girlfriend. Gemma's husband was taking online pasta-making classes so every night was an Italian feast. Rachel had moved in with her new guy, and Sarah and Dan were creating club nights in their kitchen to relive their student days. Mum was up the road, but the job now was not to kill her with the mystery disease.

Every time I called her she was 'popping' somewhere. The garden centre. The supermarket. The hardware shop.

'Mum, you are not allowed to pop anywhere!' I said.

'Of course I am. I can't stay at home all day.'

'Yes, mum, you can. That is literally what we're meant to be doing.'

'Well, that's ridiculous. I'm fine.'

And everyone seemed to be fine. I wasn't.

Attached haunted me. I remembered what it said about how avoidants tended to think they were free spirits until an emergency happened. Then our defence mechanism dropped and we needed others just as much as anyone did.

It was right.

In the first weeks of lockdown I needed people in a way that I had never needed them before. As soon as I woke up I was checking my WhatsApp groups. Throughout the day I was on Skypes and Zooms, clinging to contact.

For someone who hated neediness, this was quite a turnaround.

———

By June 2020 I had not been touched by another human in three months. I felt untethered by it. It was like I had stopped existing in some way.

I read about a study that showed parts of a mouse's brain shrinks when put into solitary confinement. The hippocampus – the part of the brain that deals with memory, spatial awareness and emotion – shrank by 20 per cent in a month.

I was a lonely mouse with a shrinking brain! No wonder I had all this time, and yet I seemed unable to do my work.

I learned that loneliness causes as much stress as being punched by a stranger, and has the same effect on our health as being obese. Lonely people are forty-three times more likely to catch a cold than people with close connections, and have 'micro-awakenings' in the night because sleeping away from others means some part of you is still on red alert for threats. It made sense of why I had been waking up several times a night. Sitting bolt upright in bed, often sweating and heart pounding.

I read that loneliness was like hunger – it was there as a sign that you had to take action. In our ancient history to be separated from the group was to mean risking death, so the pounding heart of loneliness was there to tell us to return to people as a matter of life and death.

But I couldn't. None of us could.

We were being told that we could not do the thing that our bodies were screaming for, that to do this most natural thing – be with other humans – could be fatal. To hug mum could mean to kill her.

It was awful.

The room of my own that I'd so yearned for now felt like a prison.

Daisy suggested I get a tree buddy. I found an oak in the

park and named him Dave. Before long Dave could have had me arrested for molestation.

But I didn't want to hug a tree. I wanted to hug a real person. I wanted to smell Gemma's perfume and kiss James's cheeks. I wanted to get drunk with Sarah and rock side-to-side as we hugged goodbye. I missed the closeness. I missed touch. I missed human bodies. More than missed them – I ached for them.

The difference between my life and my friends' became more extreme than ever. While I was drowning in space, they were hiding in the toilet to get a second of peace.

I called Sarah.

'I've never felt so alone in my life,' I said, my voice cracking.

'Get down from there!' she shouted. 'Sorry. I need to go.'

Daisy had spent lockdown in Brighton with her girlfriend but came up as soon as the rules allowed. We met for a socially distanced walk. We stood two feet apart with arms out in a pretend air hug.

As we walked she told me about life with her new lover. She talked about sex with a woman and how they both seemed to go in and out of the masculine and feminine roles, and how it had opened up this whole new dimension. I was eaten up with jealousy.

She asked about me and I found myself with nothing to say.

As we got to the exit of the park and it was time to say goodbye I said, 'Can I change my mind? Could we have a real hug?'

She leant in and I smelled her coconut shampoo.

'You feel so solid,' I told Daisy, my arms around her back.

'I've put on weight,' she said.

'No, I wasn't saying it like that – it's just, your body, it's so solid.'

How had I not noticed how solid bodies were before? She went to move away but I didn't let her go.

'Do you mind if we stand here a bit more?' I said, into her ear.

'Let's move out of people's way,' she said. We shuffled to a spot near a bin by the entrance to the park and kept standing there, in each other's arms. She kept hugging me and I felt something inside drop. Like some load I hadn't been aware I was carrying was taken from me. I started crying. I clung on to her.

'I'm so lonely,' I said, my voice cracked as I said it.

She squeezed me.

'I don't know how much longer I can keep living like this. On my own.'

She rubbed my back. I kept crying.

'I feel like I'm being left behind. Like you have Ann, and Rachel has her guy . . . and everyone has their families and I'm on my own and I don't matter to anyone.'

'That's not true.'

'It's how it feels. Sometimes it feels like I'm floating off the edge of the earth and nobody notices.'

'I wish you'd told me this – you kept saying you were fine,' said Daisy.

'I know.' That's the thing with loneliness, it stops you from being able to do the very thing you need to do – reach out to someone. The more alone I was, the more insecure and paranoid I became about my friends' opinions of me . . . I thought they'd think I had nobody but myself to blame for the situation I was in, because that's what I was telling myself.

'At the beginning of all this I kept telling myself that I was lucky I had nobody depending on me, that if I couldn't earn a living or if I got sick it was just me who would suffer. But then as I was saying it I realized that it's pretty fucking shit to be my age and to have nobody relying on me. Or need me.'

'So many people need you and love you.'

'Not really. I'm like an add-on. I'm nobody's main person.'

Snot was pouring from my nose now in clear, gloopy rivers. Daisy looked in her bag for a tissue. I used the bottom of my top.

'I feel like I've done everything wrong. Made all the wrong choices. I wish I wasn't the way I was. I wish I was normal and just did everything like you're meant to. I wish I'd got married, had children and had someone to share the bills with, someone to sit on the sofa with. I wish I had someone who asked me what I wanted for dinner.'

'You hate that.'

'I know. I was wrong. I wished I'd done all the things I never wanted to do.'

'You were doing other things, love. You were doing amazing things!'

It didn't feel that way now. It felt like I'd spent my life doing all the wrong things.

The most shameful thing was realizing that lockdown was extreme, but it felt like an amplification of how I'd been living anyway – alone in my box flat, typing at my box computer and spending evenings watching a box screen. It wasn't natural.

All that mattered was people.

A few days later I got a call from an old school friend. She, like me, had been single for years. She was now pregnant. Things were uncertain with the father but she was elated.

I hung up and burst into tears.

———

A family friend died of cancer. She'd spent four months on her own in hospital. Her children were not allowed in the room with her. They said goodbyes through a window.

'It's not right,' said mum. 'We wouldn't treat an animal like that.'

After that, I stopped calling people and exited my WhatsApp groups. I had nothing to say.

Instead I watched hours and hours of television. Hours and hours of people killing people in different languages, counteracted by hours and hours of *Friends*.

I stopped washing my hair and changing my clothes.

Mum told me I was depressed. I told her I wasn't.

My sister told me I was depressed. I told her I wasn't.

I called the doctor. I told him I was depressed.

I went on antidepressants.

Somewhere in my fugue state of depressed daytime sleeping and television-watching, I went on Instagram and came across a post alerting me to the fact that DEPRESSION AND ANXIETY MIGHT IN ONE WAY BE THE SANEST REACTION YOU HAVE. IT'S A SIGNAL SAYING YOU SHOULDN'T HAVE TO LIVE THIS WAY.

The person who had posted the quote said it was from a book which was 'essential reading for the times we are in'. I was sure I had it on my shelf, one of many that I'd bought without even opening, hoping as ever that the act of buying was enough to transfer the wisdom.

And there it was: *Lost Connections* by Johann Hari. The subtitle was *Why You're Depressed and How to Find Hope*.

In an act of herculean willpower I closed my laptop, where

American college kids were showing me *How to Get Away with Murder* while running around in high heels and pencil skirts, and opened the book.

It explained pretty much everything. Why humans are in the mess they're in today. Why we are so lonely, so anxious, so depressed and so stressed – even before Covid.

Johann Hari asks, 'What if depression is, in fact, a form of grief for our lives not being as they should? What if it is a form of grief for the connections we have lost but still need?'

He explains that for the vast majority of human history we existed in a tight-knit tribe of people who we slept, ate, worked and played with. Hari argues that humans are not emotionally equipped for the way we live now, either living alone or in isolated nuclear families, in which we expect one person to provide what a village used to offer us before.

The world of dog-eat-dog capitalism – where it's everyone for themselves, self-reliance is praised above all and competition is the norm – goes against everything we need as humans.

What we need, argues Hari, is community.

Every time I heard the word 'community' it made me roll my eyes. It had become another buzzword to sell us expensive yoga classes and make Facebook seem like something more than a way of harvesting our data. But that didn't mean that we didn't need real community, to get back to the village we all came from.

Hari says that we don't just need people to hang out with, but people to be 'in it' with – people with whom we have a shared goal and shared values. This identified something I hadn't been able to put my finger on – it got to the heart of what was missing, even though I had lots of friends. I was not 'in it' with others. Many of my friends lived miles away, or even in another country. We met to talk and socialize and then we went back to our own lives. In my case that meant living alone, working alone, paying bills alone.

The book told the story of a German housing development where an elderly woman facing eviction posted a note outside her front door to say she was going to kill herself. Neighbours saw the note and – for the first time – knocked on her door. They decided to band together and campaign to stop the rent increases by sitting outside their apartments and blocking the road. People who had never spoken to each other now sat together for hours, united by a common goal. The effects were life-changing.

One high-schooler who was flunking out met a neighbour who helped him with his homework, and ended up staying in school. A homeless man became part of the group, and when he was admitted to a psychiatric unit the members came together to take him out of the facility and find him a home.

One of the protestors said, 'The protests showed how weird it is – the idea that we should all sit apart from each other pursuing our own little story, watching over our own little television and ignoring everyone around us.'

Pursuing our own little story. That hit home. It was what I'd always done.

'The real path to happiness,' says Hari, 'comes from dismantling our ego walls, from letting yourself flow into other's stories and letting their stories flow into yours.'

I went downstairs and knocked on my neighbour's door. She had been texting ever since lockdowns relaxed, asking me to come down for a cup of tea, but I always made some excuse. I didn't know why I had this resistance to getting too close to my neighbours. Getting too close to anyone.

She opened the door wearing a bright-red trouser suit and matching lips, and multiple gold chains. 'Welcome, mon neighbour! Come in, come in . . .'

'Are you going somewhere?' I asked.

'Non!' she said. 'Come in, have some café.'

Stepping into her flat felt like stepping into Oz. The walls were painted yellow and lilac and were covered with multi-coloured paintings, which I later learned were all done by her. A model of ET wearing a sweatshirt sat on the kitchen table next to a bunch of tulips coming out of a vase shaped like a man's head. There were trophies on the kitchen shelves next to saucepans and a pyramid of herbal tea boxes. She saw me looking at them. 'They're for boxing,' she said.

'You're a boxer?' I asked.

'Yes!' she said.

I learned that not only was Nelly a boxer, she was also a film director, a university lecturer, and had a licence to drive lorries . . .

'I started an orchestra at NASA,' she said in passing one day. By the end nothing surprised me, including the fact that there is a Nelly Barbie and Nelly Lego.

I could not believe that this fascinating woman had been only feet away from me and it had taken nearly a year – and being stuck at home – before I got to know her.

'In London we usually ignore our neighbours,' I explained.

'I don't understand that,' she said. Nelly grew up in France to Armenian and Algerian parents. Community mattered to them.

Mum had talked about growing up in the Irish countryside where everyone supported each other. Her own mother was a nurse and was always being called on to help a neighbour with a baby being born or someone who had fallen ill. Farmers needed to help each other because they couldn't do things on their own. Mum was not just part of her family, she was part of a group of families who relied on one another. It was so far from my city lifestyle, where we could throw money at any problem – pay for a nanny, a plumber, press a button on an app to get last-minute groceries delivered by a man in a helmet who you never have to look at.

I had to relearn the old ways of weaving my life together with the people around me.

Over the coming weeks we got into a routine whereby Nelly would bang her ceiling with a broom to signal that it was time for coffee. I would go down in whatever I'd slept in and inspect Nelly's outfit – a blue ballgown, a green jumpsuit, cowboy boots, ET sweatshirts – as she made coffee and dropped some bombshell about her life.

Nelly and I spent our days together. She'd do her work calls and I'd sit on the sofa, reading and writing. One day we invited our downstairs neighbour Thomas to join us – he had moved in to the bottom of the building at the start of lockdown and I hadn't had any contact, bar signing for his parcels.

Thomas knocked on the door.

He was wearing red tracksuit bottoms, snakeskin boots and a silk shirt. He was cool in ways that I did not understand. From that day on, the three of us became a unit. Sometimes Nelly, who was also an artist, would paint as Thomas would read and I'd write. It was idyllic.

One day Nelly was painting a series inspired by ex-boyfriends. One had blue hair, yellow skin and a black hole where his heart should have been, and he was holding a strawberry.

'Why is he holding a strawberry?' I asked her.

'The question, Marianne, is why not.'

On one of our walks, Thomas said he was looking forward to getting back to the gym. 'Gay men are very judgemental,' he said. 'Screw them,' said Nelly. 'Yeah, that's what I'm hoping to do,' he replied.

When I told them how much I missed being touched they

both came in and hugged me at the same time. When they went to move away, I asked them to stay there and they did. I had now become one of those annoying hippies who wanted hugs that went on for hours.

Thomas offered to let me sleep in his bed, but I felt too shy to take him up on the offer. He sent me a picture of a woman in a black negligee with her leg wrapped around a life-sized, man-shaped pillow. 'What about this?' he asked.

I ordered a weighted blanket instead.

Sometimes we ate together, and about once a week we went down to Thomas's to watch a movie on his squishy sofa. It was domestic bliss.

At the start of lockdown I had craved someone to sit on the sofa with, and I had got it. And not just anybody – two fascinating, kind, funny human beings. Right on my door-step. And there was so much life on my doorstep, I was discovering.

I'd never had local friends, never known my neighbours or felt part of a community before. I'd spent most of my adult life moving from flat to flat, saying polite hellos to the people around me, before getting on with my life. I didn't have the time nor inclination for the inconvenience and effort that went into looking out for neighbours.

Now I did.

I joined the community Mutual Aid group and started delivering lunches to a man up the road. I didn't know what his story was, just that he didn't speak English and seemed confused every time I came to his door with sandwiches. I gave to food banks and pinned posters to trees in the rain, giving details of who people could call if they needed help.

I became a phone buddy to a blind man named Patrick. 'It's so nice to see the sun out the window,' I said on our first call. 'Um. Yes,' he replied. I wrote a list of people I knew who were also living on their own and made a commitment to call them every few days to check in. I cringed at the do-gooder I'd become.

I called Sarah. A television was blaring in the background.

'I can't take much more of this,' she said. 'I'm snapping at everyone and I hate myself for it. Dan is hiding in his shed all day . . . and the laptop is broken, and if we have to go to the park one more time I'm going to fucking explode.'

'Can I help?'

'This helps,' she said. 'Letting me vent.'

It became clear that contrary to my impressions at the start of lockdown, everyone was having their struggles. Families might not have contended with the loneliness of living alone but they had other challenges – working and homeschooling from one small London flat, for example. I read articles about the increase in domestic violence and shuddered.

I had so much to be grateful for.

20

A New Happy Ending

On Valentine's Day 2021, I woke up early. It was a Sunday and the market stalls were being put up while the rubbish collector pushed his bin. In lockdown I had spent hours watching him, engaging in the fruitless – or zen? – task of sweeping blossom that had fallen from the trees.

When the world opened up again, I thanked him. I found out he was Polish and lived in a house with three other men in West London. It took him an hour and a half and three buses to get to work every morning. He was working every day because people kept calling in sick and he didn't want the streets to be dirty.

It looked like the cheese guy wasn't there. The last time I'd spoken to him he'd said he was thinking of going vegan. 'How's that going to work?' I'd asked. 'I don't know,' he said with a shrug and smile.

A little girl on a scooter wearing an orange anorak whooshed past the fourth nail salon to open on the street, her little sister clinging on to her hood, being brought along for the ride. I smiled. The flat was warm. I'd left the heating on all night which I knew mum would not approve of – the cost! The waste! – but it was nice. The dishwasher growled as it changed into the rinse cycle and I kept watching people walk past.

Little moments – life. Happening now. Just outside my window.

A woman marched down the middle of the road wearing a powder-blue tracksuit. She looked like an angry Smurf.

Eric Fromm says: 'Love is not primarily a relationship to a specific person; it is an attitude, an orientation of character which determines the relatedness of a person to the world as a whole, not toward one "object" of love.'

At that moment I felt very loving towards the world.

I put the kettle on, opened my laptop and scrolled through Instagram. There were lots of posts about Valentine's Day, but the one I stopped to read was about being single by spiritual writer Jeff Brown:

> Not everybody is born to partner. And those who aren't should never be shamed or shunned because they made a different choice. In fact, our world would be much worse off without them. Many are here with a more individuated calling. Some are born to explore the interior realms independent of relational challenges. Others to create brilliant and bright things with little to distract them. And others have been so wounded by relationships that they feel safer and happier on their own. Whatever it is, the assumption that partnership is the measure of an actualized life is misguided. Every soul has its own path to walk. The measure of a well-lived life is whether we walk it.

As I read it, my shoulders dropped.

Every soul has its own path to walk . . .

Was I on the right path?

In the beginning of lockdown, I was sure that I wasn't. For the first time, I could really see the value of partnership and of having someone to be 'in it' with. That said, I knew couples whose relationship didn't survive the pandemic . . . so if I had been with someone, it could have been a bloodbath.

Either way, I could no longer fool myself that I didn't need people to live my life alongside.

Before lockdown I'd gotten everything I'd ever wanted – I'd written a book, lived in a small but lovely flat and had a desk with flowers on. All these things were wonderful, but in the emergency state of Covid it had become clear to me that what I wanted and what I needed were different things.

The soft animal of my body did not need a text message, nor did it need a mortgage or a marriage certificate, but it did need to be held and hugged. It needed people to make plans with, people to rely on, people who would leave me food when I was sick.

I needed to share my daily life with others.

But that didn't have to come in the form of a together-for-ever partner. In lockdown I started sharing my life with my neighbours, going in and out of each other's flats, eating, reading and watching television together, and always being able to close the door when we wanted. I had stumbled upon the most unexpected form of family.

As I sat by my desk, looking down on the street that was my neighbourhood and hearing Nelly open her blinds down-stairs, I realized that lockdown had taught me a lot. It had turned this small flat from a place I worked, watched Netflix and slept in to a home. It had taught me the value of loving your neighbours. It had also taught me about the importance of sisterhood. The concept no longer made me wince. In fact, I could see that it was the backbone of my life. It always had been, but I had never appreciated it. I had always taken the women in my life for granted.

While the men I'd met on my tantra retreats had been beautiful examples of kind, strong, open men, it was the

women I met there who I'd spoken to most days during lockdown. We had 'sister check-ins' once a week on Zoom. They
were a place where we could cry, laugh and listen. This group
became a sanctuary, along with my neighbours.

In lockdown I'd re-read *Pussy* several times. I ordered a
vibrator. I texted Daisy the link to see if she thought it was
good. 'Be careful of vibrators, they desensitize you,' she
warned. 'Get a dildo instead or try the egg!'

'I want a vibrator,' I replied.

'OK – find your bliss, love!'

I'd also ordered a few books that I'd categorize under the
term of 'female empowerment', including *Untamed* by Glennon Doyle, which had just been catapulted to bestseller lists
after Adele had raved about it.

At first, I'd hated it. I hated the breathy, melodramatic
tones to describe how women had been kept in metaphorical
cages, always pleasing. I hated the use of every moment in
her life as some epiphany.

Then I thought of Jan's teaching about how when someone
annoys us it's either a reflection of something we see in ourselves that we don't like, or something we suppress in ourselves
and wish we could be. Why was I so repelled by a woman who
dared to be happy? Who didn't parade her pain but instead her
power? Because this is what I struggled to be.

I'd started underlining.

'Women who are best at the disappearing act earn the highest praise: "She is so selfless." Can you imagine? The epitome of
womanhood is to lose oneself completely. That is the end goal
of every patriarchal structure. Because a very effective way to
control women is to convince women to control themselves.'

Oh my god, yes!

She adds: 'We do not need more selfless women . . . What
we need are women who are full of themselves.'

Yes, yes, yes.

I wanted to be FULL OF MYSELF.

I'd also read the work of radical feminist bell hooks. She wrote: 'The one person who will never leave us, whom we will never lose, is ourselves. Learning to love our female selves is where our search for love must begin.'

When I'd done all the self-love stuff at the start of my exploration into love, it had made me deeply uncomfortable. Not just the pussy stuff, but all of it. Deep down I was still held captive by the implicit and explicit lessons I'd been taught: that self-love was selfish and narcissistic.

Of course, I was wrong.

True love of oneself isn't selfish and it isn't narcissism – it is the foundation of absolutely everything. It dictates how you move through the world, how you treat others and the treatment you'll accept as reasonable from others.

But it's not easy to love yourself because it means undoing all the messages we got every day about how unloveable we are.

There isn't a moment in the day when a woman isn't being told by the media how she should look (slim and pretty), how she should behave (nice and kind and accommodating), and how she should feel (perky and grateful – 'cheer up, love, it might never happen'). We were also, of course, told how we should live (marriage and kids).

If we really loved ourselves, whole industries, relationships and possibly even governments would collapse. How many global power structures and religions are based on women not loving themselves? I was disappointed that it had taken me till my mid-forties to start waking up to this stuff – but better late than never.

A lot of self-love exercises recommend looking in the mirror. *Pussy* does, and so does Louise Hay's classic self-help book *You Can Heal Your Life*. But I didn't know how I felt about that. I could see the power in learning to love the body you live in, especially if you've spent a lifetime wishing you were taller, thinner, bigger, smaller . . . but couldn't we also be more than our bodies?

Imagine telling men that the gateway to their self-worth was to love their bodies . . . it would be ridiculous. Men are so much more than just their bodies, that goes without saying. Why shouldn't it go without saying for us too?

Beauty has been held up as the holy grail for women for too long.

For me the journey to self-love was not so much about what was going on on the outside, but what was happening on the inside. I could see that I had long been at war with myself for being the way I am: an up-and-down sort who struggles to commit and had failed to tick any of the boxes seemingly required of being a 'proper adult'.

I had been conditioned more than I'd realized to value heteronormative landmarks – marriage, kids – and to devalue myself for not reaching them. I didn't want to devalue myself any more.

In the middle of the second lockdown one of my tantra friends invited me to a Sex Magic circle to be held on Zoom. It was women only. The idea was that by using our sexual energy and pleasure we could manifest what we wanted in the world. Not so long ago it would have been a hard no, but in lockdown I said yes.

I recognized all the faces on Zoom as women who had been on Jan's tantra training. Being with them felt like coming home. These women knew me, and I knew them.

Cora sat in front of an ocean-blue sparkling wall hanging,

which matched her shimmering eye shadow and giant pendant. If Baz Lurhmann had dreamt up a spiritual sister, it would be her.

Other faces appeared on the screen, in the now-familiar Zoom boxes, and sitar music played in the background. Cora moved her computer around so that we could see her altar, which had candles burning and an engraving of a woman with a giant vulva. 'I've replaced my Buddha with a sheela na gig,' Cora said. They were going through something of a revival – recently a group of Irish artists were making them again and putting them on the side of buildings that used to be Magdalene Laundries, places where girls were sent if they got pregnant outside of marriage, places where they lived as glorified slaves while their babies were either buried or sent away.

'Shall we get into it?' she asked.

There was a pause as everyone arranged themselves, and most people moved their cameras away so that they were facing a wall.

'Take a minute to reconnect with our bodies and ourselves . . . say hello to every part of your body, with a touch, a massage or a little feather stroke. Treat every part of you with love.'

The music continued in the background. The word 'Shakti' was being sung – 'Shakti' meaning goddess.

'Feel your hands come to a gradual stop, wherever feels natural on your body.'

My hands stopped on my tummy.

'Come to a place of stillness.'

The music changed to a more upbeat piano.

'Think about what your intention is for this ceremony – whatever it is you want a bit more of in your life . . . calling in the energy of the full moon.'

I wanted more love, and more hugs.

We were reminded to breathe. The more you breathe, the more you feel.

'And when you're ready, when it feels like the walls of your temple are strong, focus on the cave inside, feeling your breath . . . your breath is like painting the walls with honey. And smile, and feel all the space inside, and we are going to make a fire in that space in your cave,' she said, like a poet.

My mind pictured it all – I was painting the walls of my body with honey and—

'So, when you're ready, start to turn yourself on . . .'

The music changed to what sounded like a woman wailing in the Sahara, but, you know, in a sexy way . . .

I kept waiting for shame or embarrassment to kick in, and it didn't.

I had lit my bedroom with candles and there was a full moon outside and there was a drum beating now—

'Feel how you can fan the flames with your breath . . .'

And I kept breathing and kept touching myself and this time it did feel like I was loving myself, celebrating myself, worshipping myself, even.

And then at some point I started to cry. Really cry. They were tears of grief for how cruel I'd been to myself, how cold and hard and scared. They were tears for the fact that I hadn't felt like I deserved this touch.

I wanted to stop, but I didn't. Instead, I kept touching myself, and soon the tears stopped and it was like the weather changed. The sun came out.

I had this strong feeling of my vagina pulsing, powerful and alive. I rested my hand there, still. I put my other hand on my 'womb space'. The mysterious, dark, awful thing that had repulsed me not so long ago now felt warm and bright and airy.

A voice from inside me said: 'Your sexuality is for you.'

Then: 'You are powerful.'

Now Cora was telling us to feel energy running from our yoni to our heart to our throat right up to the crown of our head and out into the night sky, and I really could feel it – the sexual energy running up my body.

Then the music stopped.

'Feel yourself release,' Cora was saying. 'The fire can be left to do its thing . . . let the night sky rain down on you like stardust. Holding yourself and touching yourself. Releasing everything you don't need . . .'

I lay on the bed. Surrendered.

After a few moments of silence, we were invited to come back to the camera if we wanted to. I moved my laptop to face me and looked at the other women. It didn't feel embarrassing or shameful to do this with them – it felt so natural. Their faces glowing, it felt exquisite.

I saw how beautiful women are. So beautiful.

I loved them all. I loved myself.

We gazed at each other in silence for several minutes. It was like we were swimming in a warm pool of honey together.

What an honour it was to be a woman. What a joy. What a privilege.

That week, I'd tried the jade egg again. I boiled it in a saucepan to clean it, along with three real eggs which I made into a sandwich later, and strung it with dental floss as instructed. I downloaded exercises from Layla Martin, one of which told me to hump a pillow – did all roads to sexual emancipation involve humping a pillow? – but it never quite stuck. Instead, I found other ways to allow myself to enjoy the only body that was always there for me – my own.

And the more I did that, the more I felt the truth: I was powerful.

I'd always been scared of being powerful. I thought that to be accepted I had to be quiet and nice and pretty. Self-deprecating and selfless. Malleable to whatever was needed by someone else that day.

But I was ready now. To be powerful.

What 'powerful' meant I didn't yet know, but I sensed it was to do with being unapologetic, visible, sexual. I sensed it meant dropping my people-pleasing ways and speaking the truth. I sensed it meant grabbing joy.

The next morning I dug out the lockdown paints I'd ordered on Amazon. I painted fluorescent pink flowers in a pale blue vase.

In Bloom, I wrote underneath.

I heard banging on my floor. It was Nelly giving me my morning coffee call.

'Give me ten!' I shouted down.

I ran out to the market, to Brett who sells flowers every week, rain or shine. I bought five bunches of roses and delivered one of them to Nelly, who opened the door in her dressing gown and clapped her hands when she saw them.

'My neighbooooour!' she said, hugging me.

After we had our coffee, I also delivered bunches to my sister and my mum.

'I thought you didn't have any money!' mum said when I presented her with the roses.

'They were discounted,' I lied.

'On Valentine's Day?'

'Yes.'

She raised an eyebrow and told me they were beautiful.

I FaceTimed James and Gemma. He had made me a card and I had made him one too. We waved our paper hearts in front of the screen. I told him I loved him and he told me I looked pretty.

'Do you want to hear a joke?' he asked.

'Yes please.'

'What did 0 say to 8?'

'I don't know.'

'Nice belt!'

'Very good!' I said. We beamed at each other for a second. 'I miss those cheeks so much, I wish I could kiss them.'

The screen went black as he moved his cheeks to the screen. I made a kissing sound. Then he ran off to find a car to show me, and it was just me and Gemma.

'I've been thinking about whether it's better to be single or married,' she said.

'Yeah.'

'Sometimes being in a couple is the best thing ever and sometimes it's the worst. Sometimes being single is the best thing ever and sometimes it's the worst. I think it's as simple as that. There is no better or worse way to live. Sometimes things are shite and sometimes they're good – and that's that. Also,' she said.

'Yeah?'

'We were watching *Matilda* and James said that if he had to be adopted he would be happy to be adopted by you. Just to warn you.'

'That's OK with me,' I said, delighted.

'There are many ways to be in a family,' she said.

'Yes, that's true,' I said without giving it much thought. But then I let it 'land', as they say in tantraland. 'I think I always knew that,' I said. 'But now I feel it.'

Gemma asked if there was any news from Rachel on that front.

'She's going to take a break from the IVF and just see what happens,' I said. 'But she's happy.'

The man she'd met at the gold jumpsuit party was supportive in ways she'd never experienced before, and he was on board with doing anything it took to start a family. 'If you'd have asked me what I wanted him to say, I could not have scripted it better,' she said.

That night, Nelly and I went down to Thomas. I gave him his bunch of flowers and he kissed me on the cheek. 'Thank you, darling.'

He had lit up the flat with candles and made us fondue. Fancy cheese on toast. It didn't get better. After dinner Nelly drew our portraits and we watched *My Big Fat Greek Wedding*. At one point Nelly looked up at me and said: 'You're not going to die alone.'

'What?'

'You said something before about dying alone, and I don't think you will.'

I blew her a kiss, as she drew orange spikes for my hair.

I texted the Greek to wish him a happy Valentine's Day and told him what I was watching. He replied with stickers of lips and hearts and roses. When we first met I didn't like that he sent me pictures of koalas and teddy bears. Now I loved the stickers.

We had spoken a couple of times in lockdown. 'Life is not sustainable as one person,' he'd said. 'You need two or more.'

He had spent the last few years learning how much we need the people closest to us. Without him his parents would be lost – and it had taken a pandemic for me to learn the same lesson. I could not do it alone. Nobody can. And fortunately, I didn't have to.

The Greek might not have been my happy-ever-after love story, but he was *a* love story – one of many.

For me, love had not come in the way we see in romcoms, but when I stopped focusing on a single love story, I could see that my life contained many love stories. New friends and old, neighbours, lovers, tantra brothers and sisters, my family . . .

And yet even with all this love, I often felt profoundly alone.

And as much as I loved freedom, I often felt adrift.

Perhaps that was part of the appeal of marriage and kids. When you signed up to that you had a plan for at least the next eighteen years. When you were alone, every day was a blank page. Sometimes this was wonderful and sometimes it was exhausting.

But maybe everyone is making it up as they go along. Things change, in even the most stable of lives. Marriages end. People change. Children get sick. Parents die. I remembered a friend who used to hate the phrase 'ended up', as in 'he ended up with her'. 'Nobody "ends up" anywhere,' she said. 'Everything is temporary.'

Who knew how life would unfold. Maybe I'd fall madly in love tomorrow with a man who had ten children from previous relationships. Overnight I could become a wife and mother. What a thought. Maybe I'd find myself in an open relationship, part of an intricate web of connections, or maybe I'd stay single for ever. Maybe I'd find myself raising children in some form, or maybe my writing would be the thing I put into the world. Maybe I'd live in a commune and learn to love chopping carrots and drawing up cleaning rotas, or maybe I'd stay on this street and in this flat for the rest of my days growing old with my neighbours and looking out the window at Tomasz sweeping blossom.

Whatever way it went, there would be good days and not so good days. Days of love and loneliness. Excitement and boredom. Whatever way it went, I figured it would be OK.

The last couple of years had taught me that it was not my job to *find* love, but to *be* love and to practise love. In my journal I wrote:

Love is a verb. It's not about finding the right person, it's about being the right person. Loving everything and everyone around you right now.

I didn't have to wait for a random stranger to commit to – I could commit to everyone who was already in my life.

I could also commit to myself.

Which is why I had bought myself flowers too. The white and pale pink roses sat in a vase on my desk.

As for walking into the sunset with someone . . . I didn't need to. It was already right here, setting pink and purple, orange and lilac, over the chip shop.

No Such Thing as a Happy Ending

It's now February 2024. It's been five years since I started thinking and writing about love. Lockdown is, thankfully, a distant memory.

I still see my neighbours most days. Nelly continues to wear fabulous outfits (her current obsession is leather jackets and flame-coloured Adidas) while changing the world. Thomas continues to be cool in ways that I don't understand.

As for my other friends . . . there have been changes. After eight attempts, Rachel had a baby. For the first six months she struggled. 'There is not one part of this I'm enjoying,' she said on the phone one desperate night. 'We had a lovely life and I just put a bomb in it.'

Fortunately, it got better. Months passed and her son started to smile, then laugh. They started to sleep through the night. They are now trying for another.

She does not think that having a child has magically made her life complete. 'It's not better or worse, it's just different,' she says. She still hates the narrative that you never really know love, tiredness or whatever emotion until you become a parent. 'That suggestion that, without a child, you're a fraction of the person you could be . . . it's bullshit,' she says.

Daisy consciously uncoupled from her girlfriend and has embarked on a radical experiment: being single for the first time since she was thirteen. She now lives in a dreamy flat overlooking the sea, full of fleece blankets, fleece pillows, fleece hot water bottles. She is basically living in a stuffed toy. She spends her Friday nights in hot baths, doing spells and dealing in cryptocurrency. Her biggest mission now is to get rich.

Sarah and Gemma continue to be great humans bringing up great humans, with all the highs and lows that that entails.

Sarah and Dan have decided to separate. They are still living together while they figure out how to afford two places. I sent her a link to an interview with a couple who have been living happily together since their divorce ten years earlier.

Her reply: 'No fucking way.'

But they are getting on better as friends and co-parents. We often say that marriages 'fail' – but the way they have conducted themselves looks like anything but failure.

As for me, I have lovers.

Yup. Lovers, plural.

The Catholic schoolgirl in me can't quite believe that I'm allowed to do this. To have love and freedom. Sex and space. My cake and eat it.

But it seems like I can.

I have never felt more at ease in a relationship dynamic.

One has been in my life for a little over a year. We met at a tantra workshop and both consider ourselves to be amateurs in love, lacking in experience.

'Could we maybe practise together?' I asked him after we'd spent our first weekend together. 'Practise sex. Practise communication . . .'

'Maybe,' he said, a couple of months in, 'this might be too full on, but maybe we could also practise loving each other?'

I said yes. Straight away.

If love is a verb and a skill, I need practice. If great lovers are made, not born, I need practice. And if difficult conversations and conflict are the bedrock to good relationships, God knows I need practice.

We have made a deal that we want to help each other be the fullest versions of ourselves we can be. We cheer each other on like good friends who also get naked together.

We have conversations about how we want things to be: How much do we want to talk? How often do we want to see each other? How do we feel about seeing other people? What isn't OK with us?

I didn't realize that when it comes to relationships, everything is up for negotiation, there are no rights or wrongs, as long as you are all honest with each other. Which we are.

All that practice in the workshops is paying off.

My other lover is older and wiser, more experienced in love and life. I learn from him and enjoy our time together in different ways.

I love them both, and I feel very, very loved.

There is not one part of me that fantasizes about any of us being together for ever. Not even a tiny part. I do not yearn for trips to IKEA or walks down the aisle.

None of us is trying to make the other into a version of a human we think we want or need to make our lives complete. Which is exactly what allows me to go deep. The freedom gives me huge security. It turns out that space is my love language. As soon as someone gives it to me, I fall in love.

The sex is beautiful and I still feel very much like a beginner. There is so much to learn and experience and I have the rest of my life to do just that. I am so grateful that I had the courage to go to Jan's tantra workshops. They changed my life.

It was painful to confront the gnarly feelings I had around sex but it was worth it. Getting to know myself as a sexual woman has been such an important part of growing up and it has opened up a whole new world, a world where sex is not a reward for being young and hot, but a natural and beautiful part of being human.

Sex is such a glorious thing – it's free and healthy and much more enjoyable than watching hours of Swedish crime dramas. I wish the nuns had told me this.

It is both a luxury and challenge of our time that women can explore sexuality outside the confines of relationships, and form relationships any way we want. This is not the case all around the world and it is a huge privilege that I live in a place where I can love all sorts of people in all sorts of ways.

But it took me, a Catholic schoolgirl born in the seventies, a lot of courage to explore those different ways. I spent too much time worrying about people's opinions and judgements. I was trapping myself between a rock and a hard place. I didn't want the traditional stuff, but nor did I have the guts to go after other possibilities. I didn't want to be different.

The stupid thing, of course, is that I'm not actually that different at all. More of us are living alone or finding different kinds of loves, yet we still have this hangover of the 'couple' being the norm in society. Those of us living differently need to speak up to show that this is not the case.

I have become a collector of stories about women – particularly women post-forty – who are building their lives in different ways. I follow them as if they were crumbs of bread leading me to a different place.

Two tantra friends call themselves 'monogamish', which means that the door is open if an opportunity presents itself. Mostly they don't push on the door, but the possibility allows them to feel free while also benefiting from the security of a committed relationship. They are one of the happiest couples I've seen up close. They glow.

A work friend, Rose, is in a relationship of ten years, with someone she met in her fifties. He lives in Wales and she lives in London. He has no interest in living in London, she has no interest in living in Wales. They describe themselves as 'living alone together'.

I read an article by Cindy Gallop, a sixty-something advertising guru who describes herself as a lifelong singleton who has a stable of younger lovers, many of whom she has known for years. She wrote: 'I am deliberately public about this, not to try to convince others to do as I do, but because I believe everyone should be free to design the relationship – or non-relationship – model that works for them.' She added: 'Many people are out there living lives they don't really want to live. It's all too easy to slip into the oiled grooves of what your parents want for you, what all your friends are doing, what every movie and TV show tells us we should aspire to.'

Whoopi Goldberg talked in an interview about falling into this trap: 'I thought that in order to be normal, I had to be married. So I got married, even though I knew it wasn't right. When that didn't work out I tried it again. And then again.' She continued: 'I believe in soulmates, but I don't believe that you have to have sex with your soulmate or marry your soulmate . . . I have four soulmates right now. They are people for whom I would give my life. But I wouldn't have them come live with me in my house. I don't want to marry them. They are married to other people anyway.'

Yes, Whoopi!

But I also read an article by journalist Christine Patterson, who was single all her life and found love for the first time at fifty-one. She said that being with him felt like slipping into a warm bath. It reminded me that anything can happen at any time.

I read another interview with an extraordinary human being called Anne Boden who, in her fifties, decided she was going to start her own bank. For two years she emailed people from her laptop and was basically laughed at. She now runs Starling Bank, worth several billion. She never married or had children. She happily admits that work takes up her whole life: 'I think it's important to focus on what you have rather than what you don't. I've had a great career. I've done lots of stuff. I'm proud of what we've built. I wish I could help more women understand that you don't have to conform to the stereotype to be happy, to be successful. But I've been extremely lucky. I had a childhood that was loving and supportive, but with no pressure to be anyone different.'

I was so lucky to have been brought up this way too.

One of the accusations levelled at women who don't have children is that they are cold-hearted career women. We are warned that our careers won't love us back and won't keep us warm at night. I had bought into that idea and criticized myself for how much I cared about my work. I wondered if it was all ego stuff. Vanity. Overcompensating for an empty life.

But actually, like Boden, my work has brought so much love and joy and satisfaction to my life. It was not the case that I was choosing work over love, I had just followed the path that had opened to me and poured as much into it as I could. And I got so much back in return. Some of the most meaningful moments in my life have come through my work – from writing my thoughts, meeting fascinating people, travelling the world. In some ways work has been a loyal companion, a partnership that I have always committed to.

During lockdown I read many articles exploring different ways to build a family. 'What if friendship, not marriage, was the centre of life?' asked the headline of a much-shared article in *The Atlantic* magazine. The article featured friends who have bought houses, raised children, used joint credit cards and hold medical and legal powers of attorney for each other. The author writes: 'These friendships have many of the trappings of romantic relationships, minus the sex.'

Another piece in *The New York Times*, entitled 'Mommunes', described a group of single mothers living together, sharing childcare and creating a new kind of family.

Nicola Slawson, a British writer who has written a lot about being single, announced in January that she was having a baby with her gay best friend.

I thought of my polyamorous friend from the festival. She's had her baby, who is adored by a family of three: mummy, daddy and lover. Well, former lover. I learned in lockdown that the 'lovership' – actually a word, apparently – had ended and the lover was now a friend still living in the house, and it's all perfectly harmonious.

'She looks so happy,' I said, when she posted a picture of the baby on Facebook.

'She is very loved,' said Charlotte.

What more could anybody want?

The authors of *The Ethical Slut* write: 'We want our children to be raised in an expanded family, a connected village within contemporary alienation, where there are enough adults to love them and each other, so there is plenty of love and attention and nurturance – more than enough to go around. We want a world where the sick and ageing are cared for by people who love them, where resources are shared by people who care about each other.'

Yes, yes, yes, yes, yes. I want that too and I think I'm on my way to having it.

Nelly, Thomas and I have welcomed other members into our unofficial commune gang: Gary, a musician in the next block, puts on concerts in his garden and sings up to my flat from the street when my window is open (I am serenaded!). Mary is a writer and Disney princess lookalike a couple of doors down. Susan and her son Nicholas live at the bottom of the park I spent most of lockdown walking around alone. Mum is part of the group too, she feeds Gary up with Irish stews and puts on Sunday roasts for us all. Then there's my sisters and Kem and Harry, the two brothers who run our local coffee shop, which is dubbed HQ; at any time in the day at least one of us will be in there, working, chatting, looking out the window.

For the first time in my life I feel part of a proper community. This little patch of earth is home and the people around me my family.

The question for a single person is how, practically, to build the kind of life that works for you. *The Ethical Slut* says: 'The challenge for the single slut is to find ways to deepen the intimacy in relationships that may not be life partnerships.'

Natasha Lunn's book *Conversations on Love* features an interview with Alain de Botton, who talks about asking yourself what exactly you feel you are missing by not having a partner. Is it someone to sit on the sofa with? Is it intellectual stimulation? Someone to cook with? Go on holidays with? Someone to help with practical tasks? Someone to go to bed with? To lie next to, to touch, to have sex with? Then he asks: do you really need a partner to do these things, or is there another way to meet those needs?

When I think about that question – I have people to meet almost all of my needs. I have people to talk to, work along-side, cry with, watch television with, go hippy dancing with and have sex with.

The only thing I don't have is someone to share domestic chores and bills with. Which brings me to the difficult parts of single life. When I first read Bella DePaulo on the financial cost of being single, it didn't bother me. Now it does. I won't tell you how much debt I'm in, but it's a lot. The reality is that single life is expensive, and in lockdown my mental health and productivity dropped off a cliff and I found it hard to make ends meet.

Being single in the pandemic was no joke and the worry of paying the bills all by yourself, all the time, can feel like a heavy weight even in good times. I am so grateful for friends and family who helped. I would be lost without them.

Another thing the last few years have taught me was that as a single person living alone, you need to learn how to ask for and accept help. Without someone there to witness the day-to-day of your life, people don't always spot if you are struggling. You need to tell them, to risk the embarrassment of people seeing you as a mess. I find this hard to do. I had Covid several times, and each time I insisted I was fine. Neighbours asked me what I needed and I would tell them I didn't need anything. Nelly would leave food by my door and I would feel guilty about putting her out and immediately plan to repay the favour. I could see my reluctance to rely on anyone, to be seen to be vulnerable or needy. Perhaps it was my avoidance kicking in, or perhaps this is a product of the time and culture I was born into, where independence has been prized above all.

On my fourth time of having Covid, Daisy did a giant online supermarket shop for me. I actually cried as I unpacked the items she'd bought me – tins of rice pudding, fancy chicken soup, a box of Roses Chocolates, aloe vera-infused Kleenex. I needed to feel looked after more than I'd realized. I'm now trying to make a point of saying 'yes' to all offers of help – even when I don't think I need it.

As a single woman I've spent a lot of time telling myself I shouldn't complain. I was not keeping other humans alive! I was not getting by on four hours of sleep a night! I was not going in and out of hospital with a sick child! All true. I told myself, regularly, that I was selfish and that I needed to help others more. 'Use me!' I used to say to friends. 'I'm here, I'm free!' I didn't see that I needed help too.

All friendships are based on giving and receiving, and they have to be equal to survive. This means, in my case, letting myself be helped as much as I like to help others.

At the start of my exploration of love, I wanted to be a good person, a good friend, a good sister, a good daughter, a good neighbour. Now, funnily enough, I don't really want those things. I'm done with trying to be good.

I am already good.

I came across a phrase on a podcast recently that said something like: To get to where you've always wanted to go you have to go through all the things that are stopping you.

In order to embrace new ways of living, there is lots to overcome: shame around sex, our bodies, the brainwashing that has told us we are nobody until someone 'chooses' us, or that there is only one way to be a mother and to choose not to do this makes you selfish and your life empty. I didn't realize how many messages I'd absorbed about what made a good life. I felt like a failure when I did not adhere to those norms.

Looking back, I see that my problem was never my life – it was the story I was telling myself about my life, or the one I felt the world was telling me about my life. It's time to change that story into one that celebrates the many ways there are to love and live.

I am now writing a couples' column for a British newspaper. I know! The irony of, as my sister put it, 'the most single woman in the world' writing a couples' column. Recently, a woman wrote in to say that in her forties she found herself attracted to women for the first time and she was confused about it.

The answer sex therapist Cate Mackenzie gave was beautiful: 'It often happens that people allow different parts of their sexual self to emerge later when they have the resources and confidence to take the emotional risk of trying something new, and not worrying so much about what people think.'

I like the idea that as we get older, we become freer and truer to ourselves. It made me think of the eighty-something virgin who went to one of Jan's tantra retreats. 'She had a very juicy time!' said Jan. It's a cliché but it's true: it's never too late.

As a forty-five-year-old woman with a beard and a belly (perimenopause is hitting hard), I am having the sex I've always dreamt of. The love I've dreamt of. Right now these relationships are with men, and I am open to all kinds of love in the future.

Someone else who embodies a radical freedom around relationships is Rachel E. Cargle. Her book *A Renaissance of Our Own* is about how to live life according to what you want, not the scripts the world has given you. When she started doing this, she walked away from a traditional marriage and now enjoys love with men and women.

She writes: 'I have reimagined myself as someone who can explore love and sexuality without the rules and limitations mainstream society insists on – chiefly, monogamy and heterosexuality. I have imagined myself as someone who is intentionally child-free as opposed to subscribing to a blueprint of womanhood that says that our great successes are partnership and parenthood.'

Yes, Rachel, yes!

When I read stories like Rachel's, I no longer feel like a Bridget Jones loser, I feel part of a new breed of women who are choosing to build different kinds of lives. Lives that suit them. Lives that our mothers and grandmothers were not able to choose. When we have the freedom to choose, we choose different things. For some, their deepest desire is to have children and a partner, for others, like me, our desires take us down other paths.

All paths are valid. Nothing is better or worse. I see the great beauty and richness that comes with being in a partnership and having a family. I admire the grit and grace of friends who are parents and partners. They are mature in ways that I am not. More financially stable. But just because my life is different does not make my life or theirs any less rich or interesting. Nature thrives on variety, and it's mad that we think it should be any different for humans.

A new happy ever after starts with being really honest about what we want and need. For me, sex and freedom were my deepest yearnings. I told myself that that was unrealistic and not how relationships work, but it seems to be working just fine.

Rachel wanted a child and someone to bring her tea in bed. She felt ashamed of how much she wanted someone, she thought it was unfeminist, but it was her truth. She counts herself lucky that she managed to find both of these things.

I have another friend who, the older she gets, realizes that she's just not that into people. She can go for weeks without socializing and is perfectly happy with this. She used to judge herself for being so antisocial but now she accepts that she gets joy from her animals and her garden and long walks by the sea.

Follow your bliss, as Daisy said when I got the vibrator. For some of us, our greatest love is in partnership, for others it's with animals, or trees, or friends or children. How lucky we are to live in a world with so many things to love.

At different times in life our wants and needs will be different. We must give ourselves permission to change and to make peace with the inevitable contradictions.

On one of the Jan Day retreats, we did an exercise that encouraged us to accept that two contradictory things could be true at the same time.

Instead of using the word 'but' she encouraged us to use the word 'and'.

I feel confident and scared.

I feel old and immature.

We live in a world that encourages us to be one thing but, in reality, it isn't that simple.

Recently I found my notes from this session:

I'm trying to be open-hearted . . . and I'm scared
I want to be seen . . . and I don't want to feel exposed
I love my body . . . and I sometimes feel fat and old
I deserve love . . . and that's not for me
I want to be free . . . and also I want to be close
I love sex . . . and I hold back
I love my family . . . and I need space
I'm good person . . . and I can be selfish and cowardly
I want a partner . . . and that would stop me from doing things
I want to love someone . . . and they might leave me

I want to speak my truth . . . and that might mean conflict and awkward conversations
I am powerful . . . and I put myself down

In relationships I hold a lot of contradictory feelings. One minute I really want to be with someone, and the next I don't. One minute I think I'm worthy of all the love in the world, and the next I have no idea why anyone would want to be with me.

In writing this book I kept trying to find *the* answer – the definitive answer: Is it OK to be single? Or will I be missing out?

I've come to the conclusion that there isn't one definitive answer.

Being free is wonderful . . . and so is being in a relationship.

The security of one love is precious . . . and so is the joy of many deep relationships.

Living life alongside other humans is a privilege . . . and so is having a room of one's own.

Humans desperately need attachment . . . and they also need autonomy and independence.

It's all a dance.

There are no answers. As the poet Rainer Maria Rilke wrote: 'Be patient toward all that is unsolved in your heart and try to love the questions themselves . . . Do not now seek the answers, which cannot be given you because you would not be able to live them. And the point is, to live everything. Live the questions now. Perhaps you will then gradually, without noticing it, live along some distant day into the answer.'

I just googled to see if Rilke was married. He was.

Oh, well.

———

Daisy talks about 'grieving the lives you didn't have'. She has this idea that our lives could take many paths, and there will be days when you mourn the things that could have been.

She grieves the fact that in another life she would have loved to be a mother, but in this life it's unlikely that it's going to happen. The grief that women experience when they really want to be a mother but can't have a child is one I can only imagine. And as Daisy and others have shown me, it's a grief that can be held and honoured as part of a full, happy and rich life.

Maybe in another life I could have got married and had a family. Maybe I would have been really happy. I would have been less self-obsessed, more mature. I'd have got tremendous satisfaction from loving a family.

But that person would not get to do all the things that I have been able to do – travel the world, write books or spend weeks snogging men, women and strawberries under papier-mâché dragons. She might not have had the time or energy to nurture the deep and varied friendships that made her life so rich and interesting, to act as a second mother to children who didn't keep her awake at night. She might not have had the capacity to smile at strangers and look out of windows.

I wonder if, ultimately, the best any of us can do is to trust the flow of life and to make the most of the path we are on – even if it's not the path we planned, or the path that the world tells us we should be on.

We often think of love as this desirable thing that we have or don't have, something we need to go out looking for. But maybe love isn't like that at all. Maybe love is a way of being, a deep acceptance of how life is in this moment.

Maybe love is asking us to let go of our ideas of how life 'should' be and to fully embrace what life *is*, right now, in this moment.

Maybe there is no such thing as a happy ending. If we're lucky, we wake up every day and begin again. And again. And again.

Every day a new potential love story: with ourselves, with another, with the sky, this cup of coffee . . .

With this moment.

Acknowledgements

I felt huge amounts of shame writing this book. I would wake up at 3 a.m., heart pounding and T-shirt drenched at the thought that I was writing about sex and looking at my whatever-we're-calling-it in a mirror. I stopped writing it a few times. I got back to journalism instead and enjoyed the safety of writing about other people's lives.

But I could not give up on this book. On one level because I'd spent the advance and didn't know how I'd pay it back but also because shame was the reason I had to write this. If I could play any tiny part in making single humans feel less ashamed of being single, I wanted to do that. And if I could do anything to help people feel less ashamed of their beautiful sexuality, then I had to do that too.

My friend Aisling and I did a meditation in one of the gnarly stages of writing this book, in which I imagined an alter ego. Her name was Annie and she was in a black lacy dress on stage talking about this book, exuberant and sexy. Joyous and shame-free. She was like Jessica Rabbit, if Jessica wrote a book about sex and was asked to talk about it at a book festival. I am not quite there yet but I am much closer than I was. Thank you, Aisling.

And there are many people to thank (sorry, mum*). Thank you to all my tantra friends and teachers, you showed me that another way is possible and you cheered me on through all the ups and downs of this book. Thank you Jan Day for your beautiful, scary work. I wish everyone in the world could do it.

Thank you to Mary, Preena and Helen who read early versions of this book. You showed great tact and kindness in your feedback and were so generous with your time. Mary, I will never forget the sound of you giggling while reading early pages at the table next to me, nor the hours and hours and hours of conversations where you let me benefit from your deep intelligence.

Thank you to Rachel who always believed I'd get here and who would not have been a better agent for a middle-aged Catholic school girl who was trying to write about sex. Thank you to my editors Gillian, Janice and Orla for your insights and patience. We won't go into just how late this book was but well, it was very late. Thank you Kris for getting it all going in the first place.

Thank you to my neighbours: Nelly, Thomas, Gary, Mary, Egle and Kristen, Harry, Kem, Matilda and Jamie. You are proof that it is never too late to make new friends and that doing the un-British thing of telling the truth to the question 'How are you?' pays off. Special thanks to Gary who has seen me cry more than any human should see another human cry and didn't run away. You are a real life angel.

* Mum asked me not to write acknowledgements at the end of *Help Me!* because she was fed up with 'gushing acknowledgements at the end of books' where 'anyone would think they'd prevented war the way they go on, instead of writing something that nobody is going to read.' Consider this an act of rebellion, up there with going to tantra retreats!

Thank you to all the scribblers who joined our Writing For Fun and Sanity sessions every Saturday of the pandemic. Our group was a reminder that no matter where in the world we live, we are more alike than different.

Thank you to all my friends from school, college, work, bus stops . . . I am so lucky to have you. I look forward to many more years of cheering each other on through all the different chapters of our lives.

Thank you to my mum and sisters for putting up with me even when I make life difficult for us all.

Mum – thank you for raising us to be independent women who make the most of all the options available to us.

Time to enjoy them.

Author's Note

Just because I have chosen to write about myself does not mean that my friends – and lovers – have signed up to be in a book. While the people in my life have all been very generous in telling me to write what I wanted, I have done my best to protect everyone's privacy. To that end, most of the characters in this book are composites, which means they are not based on one single person and several are from imagination.

This was especially important in the tantra chapters because at the start of all tantra retreats we all agree to confidentiality. While everything I write about happened, the details of who with have been changed. All tantra characters are fictionalised. I have written this book with Jan Day's permission and the approval of my tantra friends. Thank you so much for trusting me.

Select Bibliography and Referenced Material

'A Q&A with Esther Perel: Why is Sex So Complicated', goop podcast, 2017. www.youtube.com/watch?v=emOYH KsvUUE&t=36s

Cargle, Rachel E., *A Renaissance of Our Own* (Bodley Head, 2023)

DePaulo, Bella, 'What no one ever told you about people who are single', TEDx Talk, 2017. www.youtube.com/watch?v=ly ZysfafOAs

DePaulo, Bella, *Singled Out* (Saint Martin's Griffin, 2007) and articles available at www.belladepaulo.com

Doyle, Glennon, *Untamed* (Vermilion, 2020)

Fromm, Eric, *The Art of Loving* (Open Road, 2013)

Gray, Catherine, *The Unexpected Joy of Being Single* (Aster, 2018)

Hardy, Janet W. & Easton, Dossie, *The Ethical Slut*, 3rd edition (Ten Speed Press, 2017)

Heartbreak (The School of Life, 2019)

Levine, Amir & Heller, Rachel, *Attached* (Bluebird, 2019)

Richardson, Diana, *The Heart of Tantric Sex* (O-Books, 2010)

Thomashauer, Regena, *Pussy: A Reclamation* (Hay House, 2016)